CULTURES OF C

Biographies of carers in Britain and the two Germanies

Prue Chamberlayne and Annette King

The POLICY
PRESS

First published in Great Britain in December 2000 by

The Policy Press
34 Tyndall's Park Road
Bristol BS8 1PY
UK

Tel +44 (0)117 954 6800
Fax +44 (0)117 973 7308
e-mail tpp@bristol.ac.uk
www.policypress.org.uk

British Library Cataloguing in Publication Data

A catalogue record for this book is available from the British Library

ISBN 1 86134 166 0 paperback

A hardcover version of this book is also available

Prue Chamberlayne is Senior Research Fellow at the Open University and **Annette King** is Research Fellow at the London School of Hygiene and Tropical Medicine.

Cover design by Qube Design Associates, Bristol.

Front cover: photograph supplied by kind permission of
www.johnbirdsall.co.uk

Printed and bound in Great Britain by Hobbs the Printers Ltd, Southampton.

Contents

Dedication

To my parents, Barbara and Jack Chamberlayne, whose strong lives set me thinking about dependency and independence.

To my father, Gustav Stark, who had plans for an independent old age.

Acknowledgements

This exciting project has benefited all along from the active and generous participation of innumerable people. To the 75 carers who gave such lengthy and heartfelt interviews, and the disabled people and other household members who accommodated this process we are especially thankful.

Our special thanks also go to Holger Backhaus-Maul, Thomas Olk and colleagues at the Centre for Social Policy Research in Bremen, and Rainhart Lang and colleagues at the University of Leipzig, who not only facilitated the research but also made us personally welcome during our lengthy stays and repeated visits. We would like to acknowledge the generosity of both institutions in providing space and facilities during the fieldwork. The personal and institutional support that was extended to us on all the fieldwork visits made the stays productive and enjoyable.

We are also grateful to the assistance of the professionals, officials and community organisers in Leipzig and Bremen, who not only provided us with invaluable information and insights, but patiently guided us through the complexities of the local welfare structures, and facilitated vital links to clients and service users.

The project would have been impossible without the local interviewer-researchers in Germany. In Leipzig, the interviewers were Katrin Leonardt, Claudia Kajewski, Sina Milkün, Inge Meischner, Frauke Reinhardt and Ira Trautenhahn. In Bremen, interviewers were Jörg Baudner, Lars Brozus, Thomas Ganser, Jürgen Gerdes, Elke Grunewald, Petra Pohl and Eva Stark. As researchers on the British part of the project, Frauke Sinclair, Christine Jones and Susanne Rupp all made a major contribution.

Crucial also was the direct help and collaboration of a number of German colleagues in interview and method training, at workshops in Berlin and in London, and in individual communications. Special thanks here go to Simone Kreher from the Humboldt University in Berlin, Martina Schiebel from the Center of Social Policy Research in Bremen, and colleagues from Quatext in Berlin, notably Gabriele Rosenthal and Roswitha Breckner.

Many others have helped, most directly in the many workshops which have been held during the project and subsequently to demonstrate the method, but also in numerous local, national and international conferences and seminars, and as commentators and reviewers of the many chapters and articles which have been published on the research. Our special thanks go to colleagues in the Departments of Sociology and Anthropology, and of Human Relations at the University of East London, who have supported the project in various ways.

The writing of the book has benefited from ongoing intellectual collaboration in the Centre for Biography and Social Policy at the University of East London, in particular from the ESRC-funded seminar series which resulted in *Welfare and culture in Europe* (Jessica Kingsley, 1999), the seven-country SOSTRIS project (Social Strategies in Risk Society), and the numerous seminars and conferences which led to *The turn to biographical methods in social science* (Routledge, 2000). Of all the many participants in this work, special thanks go to Michael Rustin and Tom Wengraf. Tom Wengraf also gave invaluable help in commenting on drafts of the chapters and in helping to finalise this manuscript.

The country chapters on West Germany and Britain have also benefited greatly from Annette's work on the PhD 'Care systems in Bremen' and on the project 'Organisational factors and quality of health care: a comparison of integrated and non-integrated acute and community services' at the London School of Hygiene and Tropical Medicine. This project was funded by the NHS Executive London Region Organisation and Management R&D Programme (reference number OFHO104).

The project would not have been possible without the various grants the project received, notably from the ESRC between 1992-94 and the University of East London during 1994/95.

Prue Chamberlayne and
Annette King

Glossary

Ambulante Dienste	the German health system distinguishes between domiciliary and community services, which entail the patient or the professional being mobile (ambulant), and residential or acute hospital services.
Carer	our study mainly refers to unpaid home carers rather than to paid workers or professionals.
Caring	in this study we focus on relationships as much as tasks in caring.
Enterprises	this is the term used for former East German firms and workplaces, in which so many social activities and services were located.
Frühförderung (early development)	both East and West German systems emphasised early development for children. In the case of disability or delayed development the Federal system provides domiciliary treatments by physical and psychological therapists.
Länder	regional states, which have their own Parliaments. There are now seventeen Länder in the Federal Republic of Germany, compared with eleven in West Germany prior to unification.
Pflegewissenschaft	literally 'care science', which we have translated as 'care studies'. It denotes a new field of vocational knowledge, research and training relating to the field of residential, day, and domiciliary services.
Sozialpädagogik (Social pedagogy)	this approach to social work combines elements of counselling, culture, adult education and community work. It is centered in an developmental model of intervention and has its

own professional and academic tradition. Those
who have been profesionally trained in the subject
are called Sozialpdagogen.

Sozialstaat (Social state)	a specifically German concept denoting a corporate approach to social welfare in which the state takes a developmental role, while also mediating between stakeholder institutions. Under the system of subsidiarity many responsibilities are delegated to lower level bodies such as regions, municipalities, welfare organisations, families.
'Spring' events	the period of creative political activity between the fall of the Wall in November 1989 and the Länder elections in East Germany in March 1990. The term connects these events with the student uprisings in Prague in the Spring of 1968 (which were crushed by Soviet tanks).
Wende	the 'turning point' is a shorthand term for the social transformation in East Germany, following the fall of the GDR regime in November 1989 and German unification.
Zivildienstlëistende, or Zivis	the young people who instead of military service opt for extended medical, social or community service. Within the field of social services, Zivis tend to be assigned to welfare organisations.

ONE

Introduction

Frau Planck is a 35-year-old single mother who lives with four of her children on an estate. Her youngest son, David (aged two), who had a stroke as a baby and is tube-fed, is frequently in hospital. He receives developmental therapy two hours per week at home. Frau Planck is supposed to repeat the exercises with him three times a day.

Frau Planck left home at 15, married at 19 and had her eldest daughter at 21. Her daughter was brought up by her own parents, whom Frau Planck is currently fighting for custody. Her Turkish partner, the father of three of her children, including David, visits intermittently and gives financial support when he is in the country.

Her greatest support is a community group for younger women. Frau Planck is the only member of the group with a disabled child, but she feels accepted by them, though more generally she feels isolated and discriminated against, because of David's disabilities and because her children are half-Turkish.

Interview, Bremen 1992

Mrs Elliot, who is 60, cares for her 29-year-old grandson Michael, who has learning disabilities and is now developing progressive blindness and epilepsy. He attends a daycentre five days a week.

Having emigrated from Jamaica in the 1960s, Mrs Elliot's family has lived in London's East End for most of their lives. When her daughter became pregnant at 14, Mrs Elliot kept the child. Her daughter then emigrated to the United States in the early 1970s. In the 1980s, Mrs Elliot divorced her husband.

From her wages as a home machinist, she struggles to support herself, her grandson and (until her recent death) her mother. She works long hours to make ends meet, and does not get out a lot. A small network of friends keeps her company while she is working, and she has good links with the local carers' group and with Michael's day centre. She and Michael have a close relationship and, especially since her daughter recently came back to Britain and now lives with them, Mrs Elliot sees no need to change her arrangements in any way.

Interview, East London 1994

Frau Hager is 59, single and uses a wheelchair. She had a brain tumour removed some time ago which caused serious degrees of paralysis, some of which may be returning. She cares for her mother, who is 90, blind and frail. Frau Hager coordinates the assistance which she and her mother receive from various agencies, and spends a great deal of time keeping her mother company and helping her.

Mother and daughter have always been close, but have lived independent lives. Frau Hager was a book editor, which allowed her to structure her work and her caring around her own disabilities. Since unification, she can no longer find work. She receives an invalidity pension, but would have preferred to keep on working. She attributes her situation to German unification as much as to her own or her mother's deteriorating health. Through a large circle of friends, she keeps up her many social interests and, despite financial and health restrictions, hangs on to her sense of independence.

Interview, Leipzig 1992

Our approach

Case studies focus on the mystery which lies at the heart of social inquiry, the mutual shaping of individual lives and social structures. In this book, we use the lived experience of individuals as a way of exploring the nooks and crevices of particular situations and personal responses, and for tracing how those in turn are shaped by the wider structures of specific social systems. We also invite readers to weave back and forth between identification with the individual case studies and more distant and abstract levels of comparison and theorisation. Moving between closeness and distance, and between particularity and abstraction is mutually enhancing, as we hope the cameo portraits above suggest. The portraits already embody three key dimensions of our inquiry: the intensity of personal dilemmas within caring; the individualised nature of particular circumstances and personal relationships; and the embeddedness of each situation in a decisively 'West' or 'East' German or 'British' context.

Our research subjects are carers, mainly but not exclusively women, whose main life focus has for varying periods of time centred on a seriously disabled family member[1]. They are welfare subjects who have been faced by a life-changing challenge. How carers meet this situation, the biographical resources they bring to it, the public ideologies which bear upon them, the extent to which they avail themselves of formal and informal external resources, and their confidence and competence to confront official diagnoses and decisions, is the subject of our inquiry. How carers come to terms with and negotiate the restrictions of their situation, and how they deal with the issues of power and dependency in relationships of such proximity and inequality, are also our concern.

From the detail and variety of the case studies we can discern how cultural and social patterns relating to particular welfare regimes produce typical and recognisable adaptations to the challenge of care. These responses may be at odds with official policy – indeed, it may be a perverse effect of welfare systems that the most vigorous and creative responses to them are necessarily in some sense oppositional or resistant. Welfare systems are, after all, bureaucratic authorities and forms of service, and are widely perceived as such. In taking account of the life experiences of carers, and the personal, cultural and social resources out of which informal caring is constructed, we are assisted by the instruments of the biographical approach. From the personalised accounts these instruments yield and the forms of analysis they provide, we can trace the history and cultural embedding of individual actions and pathways.

Welfare regimes

How best to characterise formal welfare systems remains an evolving and contentious art. Our broad social and cultural approach exemplifies these difficulties, as does our focus on social service and health contexts, on the interfaces between public, social and private spheres, and on experience and process. Our emphasis on the contextualised dynamics of caring signifies a new stage in the development of comparative social policy.

Whatever their limitations, mainstream characterisations of welfare regimes – which tend to focus on social security systems – have direct implications for gender patterns and caring practices. We find a useful starting point in Titmuss' (1975) categorisation of three models of welfare: industrial achievement, residual and institutional. In this schema, West Germany[2] exemplifies the 'industrial achievement' model, distributing rather generously on the basis of merit, work performance and productivity, acting as a 'handmaiden' of the economy. This system is corporatist, giving pride of place to occupational groupings and to partnership agreements between the state, the banks and industry. Its federal system also cedes considerable regional autonomy. As Lewis (1992) points out, this is a 'strong breadwinner' model which prioritises male earnings and leaves women's roles centred in the family, with few incentives to married women's employment and rather little public provision for nursery age care. British welfare, by contrast, has since the 1980s been based on the individualistic 'residual' model, which stands aside from the economy and minimises forms of state support in order to give free rein to the market. This system also relies on the strong breadwinner role, with the difference that its low wages often necessitate both partners working and cause family stress and breakdown, resulting in a high incidence of single parenthood. The 'institutional' model, which is based on principles of collectivism, is more comprehensive and egalitarian than its counterparts. Scandinavian welfare systems and Britain's earlier postwar welfare state are the main references for this model. Its nearest approximation in our study is the East German system of state socialism. In this 'weak breadwinner' model, there is widespread public support for family functions; women are treated independently and tend to be fully employed.

The breadwinner approach to policy analysis, which draws attention to gender and family ideologies, shares the employment-centredness of the welfare regime models. It underplays many wider aspects of sexual politics and citizenship rights. Comparisons of corporatist, liberal and social democratic welfare regimes by Esping-Andersen (1990) and Leibfried (1993) also centre on social security aspects, neglecting health and social service structures. There are, however, strong connections and disjunctions between these policy areas which are crucial to the lived experience of the actors in our study. West German emphasis on productivity leads to bifurcation between state and occupationally-based insurance on the one hand, and locally and often church-administered assistance and welfare on the other. Yet care benefits are relatively high and comprehensive in the Federal system, and domiciliary services more systematic and better funded than in Britain, despite a common pattern of administrative fragmentation. In Britain social services have been diverse and inconsistent, with community care policies caught between centralising and local pressures. East German prioritisation of production led to the neglect of local and residential services, but gave rise to training and jobs for the less severely disabled, a strong system of workplace identities and mutual self-help through informal social networks. Such differences in service structures and levels of provision escape the mainstream welfare models, but are crucial to comparisons of caring contexts.

Culture

In our study, patterns of informal caring emerge not as the direct product of official welfare systems, but as a cultural phenomenon in their own right. 'Culture', in our usage of the term, interweaves an analysis of action (both intended and actual), meanings (ideologically received and more personally derived), and patterns of social resources and relations. It centres on the life worlds of carers, meaning a contextualised account of their experiences, drives and motivations. For a wider discussion of sociological approaches to culture, see Berger and Luckmann (1967) and Geertz (1975). For a discussion of cultural approaches to the analysis of welfare see Chamberlayne et al (1999) and, less directly, Williams et al (1999) and Titterton (1992).

In our view, when structural determinants produce consequences for identities, everyday strategies and social relationships, then a cultural pattern has emerged, particularly if it has an enduring and reproducible character. In considering contexts we distinguish the *private* level of personal and family situations, the *social* level of informal networks, and the *public* level of structures and resources. In fact these levels are closely intertwined: the gender patterns within caring, including patterns of partnership among carers, are socially as well as personally determined; patterns of employment among carers, or of housing size and layout, contain dimensions of individual choice as well as public policy. As we have already indicated, patterns of informal networks are in many ways a response to public regimes.

Treating welfare subjects not only as constrained and enabled by, but also as creative of, the social conditions in which they exist leads to a cultural approach to welfare. The actions of welfare subjects are by definition culturally influenced, by issues of gender and generation, by attitudes to disability and family privacy, and by patterns of mutual cooperation and sociability. All these involve wider cultural patterns and attitudes than can be attributed to specific welfare regimes.

Moving between personal, social and public dimensions of caring inevitably leads to some fluidity in our definitions of 'cultures of care', especially since we are making comparisons and connections between welfare regimes and carer strategies. On the one hand, we are seeking to characterise the dynamics of informal caring in each of the three societies studied, identifying the caring strategies which seem most typical of each welfare context. On the other hand, as we move beyond the analysis of caring in each particular society to focus on the implications of the study for new thinking in social policy, we shift to the social and policy ingredients which seem most to promote wider outside and civic engagement among carers. In advocating a new, more cultural approach to social policy we are necessarily transcending discussion of any welfare regime as it presently exists.

Thus the emphasis shifts within the book from a focus on caring within particular welfare regimes in the early chapters to a greater emphasis on comparisons of carers irrespective of regime in the later chapters, whether at the level of individual biographical strategies or at the level of the informal social sphere. This allows a discussion not only of the features of particular regimes, but also of possible transnational issues and developments, both in community care and in more general aspects of social policy. These more general aspects include gender relations within caring, and changes in the constitution of meanings of private, social and public spheres in the context of (post)modernisation.

History

However varied the ages of our carers, the length of their caring experience, and the life span covered in their accounts, all interviewees convey a certain historical depth, since every account refers to the past as well as the present and future. The carers speak of experiences which stretch back in time – to the 1950s among older people – so that the time horizons of the book span several decades of the postwar period. Albeit partially, the study represents lived experiences of the three welfare systems across this span of time. In the case of East Germany, the project documented the workings of the state socialist model of welfare through the biographies of its subjects. In many senses this is a 'new' portrayal of that society, since very little ethnographic or qualitative research was conducted under the state socialist regime. The study depicts two changes of welfare regime: the dramatic change in East Germany since 1989 from state socialism to the West German Federal system of subsidiarity and the social state, and the decisive switch in Britain in the 1980s from social democracy to neo-liberalism. It also traces significant changes within the West German system in that period. The study of East and West Germany has given us 'new eyes' with which to interpret welfare developments in Britain.

Our second use of the wide time span in the interviews is to consider caring careers and trajectories, how carers incorporated caring into their prior lives, and whether doing so involved processes of continuity or change. This temporal dimension is a distinguishing feature of the biographical method as compared with other qualitative approaches.

Reader pathways

Readers with prime interests in comparative analysis, the social professions, community work and policy making, or methodology will approach this book with their own quests, and some may want to select certain strands of analysis.

Comparativists may be most interested in the book's injecting of experience into the abstract models which predominate in comparative social policy, and its enlivening of such concepts as German subsidiarity and Anglo-Saxon neo-liberalism. Some may home in on the relatively neglected model of state socialism in East Germany, which is described in some detail. As enchantment with market liberalism in Central Europe diminishes, and as European Union (EU) membership for Poland, the Czech Republic and Hungary becomes more imminent, so the legacies of state socialist models of welfare regain interest. The swiftness of East German incorporation into the western market model has been remarkable. The remaining divisions between the 'two Germanies' have been equally so. Rather than second-guessing which aspects of East German culture will survive, our interest focuses on several aspects of the cultural dynamics of East German society which seem relevant to new developments in social policy.

Health and welfare professionals and educationalists may be more drawn to the personal dynamics of caring biographies and what the different patterns imply for intervention strategies. Carers' biographical work in making sense of the experience of caring can be greatly helped by professional support. Professional interpretations and repertoires of intervention in caring situations can also be enhanced by attention to welfare contexts and social structures. The interventions we call for work across and within personal, social and public spheres.

Community workers and policy makers may like to focus specifically on our analysis of the informal sphere. For us, caring offers a doorway to the study of informal systems of welfare, to the extending of comparative social policy to that level, and to a transcending of the welfare regime approach. Recent social policy discourse in Europe and in Britain emphasises the mobilising and strengthening of social capital, capacity building, active welfare and the third sector. Realisation of these concepts presupposes an understanding of resources and processes within the informal infrastructures of society; politicians, policy makers, professionals, researchers and service users need to be able to think and speak strategically about the informal social sphere. This study's exploration of the social relations and dynamics of informal caring in three societies aims to contribute to such awareness and discourse.

Some readers' prime interest may lie in the methodology of the research, in particular the pioneering use of biographical methods in a three-way comparative study. Recent years have seen an expansion of interest in subject-centred, qualitative methods, and in narrative, life history and biographical methods. Our particular turn to the biographical-interpretive method forms part of a much wider phenomenon. Readers may be interested in the particulars or in the more general qualitative character of the method we have used. Detailed discussion of our procedures is minimal here, since it exists elsewhere (Social Strategies in Risk Society (SOSTRIS) Working Papers 1-9, see especially Breckner 1997; Chamberlayne et al, 2000; Wengraf, 2001). Our focus lies rather in demonstrating the use of biographical methods as a research tool breaking new ground in social theory, social policy and comparative analysis.

New welfare perspectives and case study analysis

New orientations in social policy towards active welfare and the mobilising and strengthening of social capital emerge in a range of political currents. For example, emphasis on more active participation in welfare comes simultaneously from new social movement politics, neo-liberalism and Third Way thinking. It is central both to New Labour's 'welfare to work' programme in Britain, and Chancellor Schröder's 'activating social policy' in Germany. In the latter, a more personalised and interactive case study approach in social assistance procedures is supposed to create a 'trampoline' towards fuller participation in society (Breckner et al, 1999, p 65).

The idea of building more directly on the informal infrastructures of social capital sits at a similar confluence of political currents, both internationally and within Europe. Ackers (1999) wryly comments that increased reliance on the informal sphere is the corollary to welfare retrenchment (p 73). Yet the concept of social capital resonates as much with the radical tradition of mutual self-help as with the more conservative philosophy of communitarianism (Frazer and Lacey, 1993). We adopt Putnam's (1993) definition of social capital as the capacity to mobilise support and resources in the informal sphere, based on norms of reciprocity and networks of civic engagement (p 167). The term is widely used in British urban regeneration policy as a hidden feature of local cultures, which should be recognised and strengthened (see also Gamarnikow and Green, 1999).

The shift in social theory towards emphasis on subjective agency and interrelationships between individual action and social structure has been curiously slow to produce empirical work, and slow to reach the discipline of social policy. As we discuss in the two volumes *The turn to biographical methods in social science* and *Welfare and culture in Europe* (Chamberlayne et al 1999; 2000), the rising popularity of biographical research tools may well lie in their aptness for exploring subjective and cultural formations, and tracing interconnections between the personal and the social.

For us, one of the excitements of encountering biographical methods has been the discovery of ways of linking separate currents in sociology, such as the study of personal and social meaning and interactive relationships (in phenomenology and social interactionism), with wider social structures and power relations (in structuration theory) (see Holstein and Gubrium, 1994). A focus on local and specific details within case studies can illuminate the complex and fluid ways in which power operates. Structural forms become accessible through the analysis of contextualised personal experiences (King, 2000, p 310). Others have argued similarly in recent years. Gottfried (1998) invokes the Gramscian philosophy that subjects' praxis reveals the 'real' conditions of their existence (p 457), arguing that: "an excavation of the operational logic of everyday life can uncover the active constitution of gender and class in practice" (p 452). Bell and Ribbens (1994) maintain that it is through the study of everyday life that the relationships between structure, consciousness and action can be explored.

That case study methods could be used to investigate social contexts in a systematic, comparative fashion was something we discovered through the *Cultures of care* project (King and Chamberlayne, 1996). We only came across the biographical interpretive method as we were embarking on the project, realising that its narrative method would be a good way of exploring uncharted aspects of carers' situations and experiences. We also knew that German colleagues who used the method employed a theoretically grounded procedure of interpretation, which struck us as an advance on the intuitive approach of much qualitative research in Britain. As we set about analysing particular cases, however, with all their personalised detail, we were not at all sure that we would arrive at structural comparisons. Despite the more widespread use of the biographical-interpretive method[4] in Germany, such methods had not been used in comparative investigations of welfare. Studies in Germany which used the method focused on what, from a British point of view, might be considered middle-range theories of life course 'careers', and changes in social worlds, social milieus and social movements (Apitzsch and Inowlocki, 2000, p 64). To our delight, in comparing East and West German cases, 'system effects' sprang into view, and we realised that through the case studies we could see the way in which individual lives are lived through particular systems, and particular systems lived out in individual lives. Using biographical methods comparatively therefore represented a new point of departure, from both German and British standpoints.

Gender issues

Our research grew out of and builds on a strong body of feminist work on caring, much of which pioneered later developments in sociology, as in methodology and in theories of the body and of the emotions (Shilling, 1997; Duncombe and Marsden, 1993). Our contribution to gender analyses of care lies in bringing context into caring, exploring its intersections with the public, social and private spheres, and probing more deeply into personal and family dynamics in caring situations (Jones and Rupp, 2000).

Insistence on the subjective dimensions of caring activities and relationships, and boundary-breaking uses of small-scale qualitative methods were hallmarks of feminist work in the 1980s and early 1990s. Graham (1983, p 29) emphasised the need to transcend the gap between treating caring as work, which was common in social policy, and regard for psychological bonds within the caring relationship (see also Finch and Groves, 1983). Ungerson's (1983) work explored "largely unarticulated" social rules and the complexities of "hidden and unrecognised" feelings in caring. Her attention to feeling states also drew on "my own psyche as the generator of research ideas" (p 77). Such exploration of identification and empathy between researcher and research subject later became more widespread (Ribbens and Edwards, 1998). Lewis and Meredith (1988) explored the intertwining of obligation and affection in mother-daughter relationships in caring, and others tackled the gendered nature of issues of power and dependency in familial caring (Parker, 1992; Finch, 1989; Ungerson, 1987; Qureshi and Walker, 1989). Twigg and Atkin (1994) focused on dynamics between professionals, informal carers and disabled people. American writers such as Tronto (1993) and Moller Okin (1991) summarised this bridging of practical, moral and emotional dimensions as 'the ethic of care'. Despite feminist analysis of welfare as the outcome of a constant redefining and repositioning of public and private spheres (Pateman, 1989), there has been little empirical emphasis on structural and cultural contexts of caring. An exception was the study by Finch and Mason (1993) on the way carers actively negotiate moral rules in a process of working out 'the proper thing to do'.

Postmodern perspectives, demanding a more culturally and socially differentiated approach, brought criticism of the anglo-centrism and middle-class bias of much of the work on caring (Graham, 1991). Ungerson (1987, p 143) had already pointed to the resistance of some women to taking on caring roles (see also Thompson, 1995), and more attention was paid to racial and ethnic dimensions of caring situations and experiences (Atkin, 1991; Ahmad and Atkin, 1996). Meanwhile, members of the disability and independent living movements criticised the very concept of caring, and the oppressive nature of dependency-inducing forms of family care for disabled people (Morris, 1993, p 34).

In the more Europeanised research era of the 1990s, feminist work oriented to debates on citizenship and on payments for care (Knijn and Kremer, 1997; Ungerson, 1997; Hervey and Shaw, 1998). Within such policy debates, carers are variously treated as an endangered species, a marginal group excluded from labour market rights and protection, and an emblem of continuing gender inequality in the home and in employment. Payments for caring, pension credits for childcare, and leave for family reasons are all potent ways of giving a public profile and social value to previously invisible reproductive work. Feminists also argue for a gender-sensitive approach to citizenship, which is less individualised and takes account of dependencies, and which serves women's needs for personal growth and autonomy (Knijn and Kremer, 1997; Orloff, 1993).

Emphasis in feminist analysis on women's emancipation has been challenged in recent years on two fronts, firstly by a shift from women's studies to gender studies, which removes the primary focus away from women, and secondly by technological and labour market developments. It may be that gender patterns in relationships between the public and private spheres are fundamentally changing, however slowly, and that meanings of the public-private divide vary among societies and among individuals, much more than feminist analysis has allowed. Our study shows the huge cultural shift in women's ways of relating to the public and private spheres in the German Democratic Republic (GDR), following three generations of full employment of women. The employment of women, part-time and flexible forms of employment in the service and information economies, and long-term unemployment all radically affect home-employment and gender relations (Hochschild, 1989; Kemmer, 2000). More varied and flexible home-employment relations, especially in a context of computerised homeworking, challenge the image of home-based work as narrowly confined within the domestic sphere. Balbo (1987), speaking of women in developed western welfare systems, argues that through their skills in mediating family relationships, informal networks, and a range of health, welfare and housing services, women have been catapulted from the periphery to the centre of society, so relevant are such skills to present-day labour markets. On the other hand, welfare retrenchment under the impact of neo-liberalism exerts pressures towards the reprivatisation of welfare problems, and pressures towards 'family-alone' solutions are growing continually. In our study, this tendency is most evident among British carers.

The comparative nature of our study offers some insights into how caring is being affected by counterposed tendencies towards tighter and looser gendering of roles. Key factors include patterns of women's employment and different gender regimes in the three societies studied, partner roles, attitudes of social professionals, and differences between age and occupational groupings, all of which vary between the three societies. We explore the dynamics of the 'Cinderella situation', which certainly exists. But generally, our findings support the Balbo (1987) thesis, showing that carers are strongly affected by modernisation processes and are often drawn out through caring into wider public engagement. We compare situations in which carers choose to take the sole responsibility of caring upon themselves, or are pushed to do so by deteriorating services, with situations in which carers gain greater access to the outside world through caring and increase their social competences.

Partner roles emerge as significant features of these different modes of caring, and the male carers in the study provide useful examples of differences between men's and women's ways of transcending the public–private divide. Men play a larger part in the study than is apparent at first sight. Husbands often figure in the accounts of women carers, some of the individual interviewees were men, and some interviews were undertaken by a couple.

The social sphere

The public worlds of employment and welfare services shape caring situations and strategies, as does the private sphere, in which we include personal and family dynamics and expectations. But between these poles lies the sphere of networks and associational life, which we regard as equally crucial in mediating carers' relations with the outside world. It is often through the filter of such informal cultures that the meaning of employment for identity or carers' capacities to negotiate with services are defined. Riley (1988) stresses the significance of the enmeshment of women's lives in the social sphere of public health and reform in the 19th century, both as subjects and objects of reform, as a pathway to wider public life. Riley's study provided an important cue for us, since gender dimensions are curiously neglected in much of the literature on civil society and the informal sphere (for example Rosanvallon, 1988; Putnam, 1993; Hirst, 1994).

Working from our case study material, we explore in each society the pattern and culture of infrastructures available to carers beyond the door of their home, and what meanings and motivations were involved in their strategic use or rejection of them. We particularly distinguish networks which expand support for the private sphere of caring from those which draw carers out into a wider world of social contacts and civic engagement. Through this we aim to contribute towards a more differentiated and gendered understanding of the informal socio-cultural sphere.

Broadly speaking, our findings are that in West Germany the pull is overwhelmingly towards the private sphere; carers are almost pressganged by social and family expectations into full-time service and have few outside connections. Those who escape these pressures are more marginally positioned in relation to traditional family structures. The British carers are involved in a denser mesh of social connection, particularly when their disabled children are young. Later in the life cycle the unreliability and indifference of services, together with an absence of professional support in making difficult decisions, propel them back into personal solutions. In Britain there is a less compelling ideology towards a home orientation than in West Germany, and husbands, who tend to favour outside solutions, are more directly supportive in caring tasks and decisions. In East Germany the cultural habit of using full public childcare provision and of women working removes the overt pressure to be home-based. Carers' everyday life-world experience of finding advice through informal networks and sympathetic professionals propels them towards outside solutions. Later in the book we move beyond these national comparisons in a discussion of what seem to be key ingredients and dynamics of a more outward-oriented approach to caring, drawing on features of more outwardly-oriented strategies in all three societies. Chapters five and six and the conclusion advocate a cultural approach to social policy, which would support biographically sensitive and imaginative work among carers and bring all the social benefits associated with outward-orientedness and enhancement of social capital.

Background to the project

The fieldwork on which this book is based was conducted in 1992-93 in West and East Germany, and in 1995 in Britain. Its was funded by the Economic and Social Research Council (ESRC) for 1992-95 (*Cultures of care* project, R000 233920), and then by the University of East London for 1995-97. This comparatively extensive research time scale allowed us to participate in the new Europeanisation of social policy research. It was a period in which dialogue and communication among social scientists took a quantum leap, through Erasmus student exchange programmes, conferences, observatories, thematic networks and collaborative research projects.

The initial project of comparing caring in East and West Germany was conceived in the early stages of German unification, when the two parts of the reconstituted country were faced with the task of getting to know each other. Academic expertise in Britain was likewise restricted to one or other of the two Germanies. The *Cultures of care* project aimed to contribute to the bridging of this knowledge gap. Annette King, who grew up and did her initial higher education in West Germany before moving to Britain, had no knowledge of East Germany. Prue Chamberlayne, who had visited West Germany in her school years and as an undergraduate of German, had more recently focused on East Germany, which she had visited regularly since 1987 as a researcher. Together we could usefully supplement each other's knowledge.

Our background knowledge and experience of East and West Germany and our language capacities were a prerequisite of using the 'safari' model of comparative work, in which one set of researchers undertakes the fieldwork in various settings, and becomes acquainted with local researchers and with local social science literature. This method has the great advantage of mediating social scientific work among societies (Chamberlayne and King, 1996, p 103). More usually, European comparative research is conducted through networks of national collaborators, coordinated by an observatory which remains distanced from the research field. In our case, prolonged fieldwork visits allowed time to involve local interviewers in initial processes of analysis, and for wider local discussion of the research with friends and in academic seminars and conferences. Through Erasmus and previous research visits and contacts we had extensive links with social scientists and with German social science literature (Annette King started her PhD *Care systems in Bremen* in 1991).

The fieldwork and interview method

As indicated, we came across the biographical-interpretive method in the run-up to the research and were excited by the way it seemed to answer problems we were encountering at the piloting stage. Semi-structured questions were failing to gain depth or to generate a new perspective on our research questions concerning public–private relations in caring situations. We felt that if we really wanted to understand the social constitution of caring, we had to find a technique with the capacity to work across the boundaries of personal and social, and private and public aspects of caring[5].

Having encountered the biographical-interpretive method, our interviews used a modified version of the open narrative technique developed by the German sociologist Fritz Schütze, which is part of the research approach developed by Gabriele Rosenthal and her colleagues (Rosenthal, 1993). Our opening prompt asked carers to talk about their experience of caring, how it had developed over time, what forms of support they had had or might have wished for, and what caring meant to them personally (see Jones and Rupp (2000, p 277) for a critical discussion of this opening prompt). We stated that we were interested in their experience and would not ask questions until later[6]. Our aim was to allow interviewees to develop their experiences according to their own frame of reference, without undue direction by the interviewer. This freestyle phase in the interview was followed by questions about the account, clarifying what had been said, and about themes that had not been covered in the initial narration. Questioning for purposes of deepening, clarifying and gap-filling continued in the second interview.

While we conducted some of the interviews in Germany ourselves, most were undertaken by five or six local interviewers in each of the two research localities – Bremen in West Germany and Leipzig in East Germany. Interviewers were identified through local academics, and tended to be postgraduate students or researchers from the fields of sociology, education or psychology. One interviewer in East Germany was a professor, recently made redundant through the process of unification. The training was conducted in two or three workshops in each city and at one joint workshop, and was led by research consultants Simone Kreher from Humboldt University and Martina Schiebel from the University of Bremen, who were experienced in biographical methods. They introduced the interviewers to the general principles of the method, and trained them in narrative interviewing and in the first steps of analysis. The interviewers wrote fieldnotes, and undertook some initial data analysis, such as the listing of biographical data and sequentialisation of the text (see below and Wengraf (2001) for a more detailed account of these procedures). For the British part of the study, Frauke Sinclair conducted the background research and fieldwork in two contrasting boroughs of London, while Susanne Rupp and Christine Jones did the analytical work and writing up[7].

In Leipzig and Bremen, the project began with interviews with officials from the main welfare agencies, giving access to local organisers of domiciliary services, with whom interviews were also held. In the absence of systematic lists of carers, organisers typically offered one or two known to them. Contacts were also made through self-help groups and children's homes. The interviewers assisted in finding interviewees, including through personal contacts. In Britain, Frauke Sinclair visited carers' representative groups and interviewed local authority development workers, making presentations at carers' meetings to find interested participants. Local carers' organisations provided the main point of access to interviewees.

In all, interviews were conducted in 24-26 households in each city, mostly twice, for a period of one or two hours each. Interviewees were selected on the grounds of variation in terms of age, sex, ethnicity, occupation, education and caring relationship (see Appendix 2), and we deliberately sought people covering a wide range of disability and chronic illness. The sample included carers of parents and of partners, both younger and older, and carers of children of varying ages. About a quarter of the interviewees were men – five in West Germany, eight in East Germany, and six in Britain. Of these, 13 were men caring on their own, rather than in a couple. Four of the British carers were from ethnic minorities; despite considerable efforts we were unsuccessful in gaining access to such carers in West and East Germany.

Method of analysis

All 76 interviews were transcribed and for each a case profile was written, giving an overview of the particular case; 24 interviews were analysed in depth, eight from each society. The selection of interviews for in-depth analysis was based on two principles. One was the pairing of cases between the societies according to external features: we chose pairings of older carers who might be caring for spouses or adult children, middle-aged carers who might be caring for spouses or for children making the transition to adulthood, and parents caring for young children. The second principle was theoretical sampling (Glaser and Strauss, 1967): having analysed one case in each society, we selected further cases which seemed similar or contrasting in terms of emergent themes. The initial emergent themes, derived from the interview profiles, were ways of mobilising resources, issues of power and control, and ways of coming to terms with disability.

Key features of the method of case reconstruction lie in distinguishing and then analysing the interplay between two dimensions of the interview: the practical life events and the way people talk about them. These two strands are often referred to as the lived and the told story. Making sense of the experience of caring during the interview involves the carers in an active process of reflection and biographical work, as it has at many times in the past. The analysis aims to reconstruct this process of self-theorising. The resultant case studies go beyond the self-presentation of the carers, because of the interpretive work of the researchers. Readers will also be involved in their own critical and imaginative work, drawing on their own life experience and making their own inferences. This dynamic interpretive work, with its emphasis on action and latent meaning, distinguishes the biographical-interpretive method within the broad and rich range of life history, oral history and narrative approaches[8].

Our method of interpretation therefore begins by a separate analysis of the objective biographical events in the life, as much as these are mentioned in the interview account, and continues in an interpretation of the structure of the self-presentation, as this is revealed in the construction of the narrative. These two forms of analysis adopt a procedure of sequential hypothesising about what meaning any datum could have or have had for the narrator and what could happen next, in the life or in the story. Each form of analysis starts off in a three-hour workshop, in order to broaden the spectrum of interpretations and the base of contextual knowledge. Hypotheses are confirmed or disconfirmed as the analysis continues, the approach emphasising active patterns of selection and leading to structural or overall hypotheses concerning emergent strategies. Profiling what could happen as well as what does happen highlights choices, both at key junctures in the life and in the telling of the story. In the analysis of the narrative account, much attention is paid to whether a past, present or future time perspective is being adopted at any particular point, and to shifts in self-evaluation over the life course.

Emergent structural hypotheses or themes concerning the structuring of the life and the structuring of the story are then compared and elaborated in a case reconstruction, which combines an outline of the practicalities of each caring situation with an interpretation of the carer's life course and approach to caring. This analysis is written up as a case study.

The process of comparing and theorising from cases and making comparisons across societies follows the principles of grounded theory (Glaser and Strauss, 1967). This involves staying close to the detail of the case study material, with its 'thick description' of the social context (Geertz, 1975), but also weaving to and fro between this detail and more abstract levels of analysis, and between the individual situation and the structural context. Scheff (1997) describes this process of relating the smallest parts to the largest wholes as "shuttling up and down" the part/whole ladder (p 58). Unlike the systematised stage of individual case analysis, the comparing of cases proceeded somewhat intuitively and anxiously, as we have indicated above. The prospect of comparing such multifaceted cases at first seemed daunting. In fact, by presenting two separate and contrasting cases in some detail, and carefully considering their similarities and dissimilarities, clear patterns emerged which could be extended, qualified and developed into typologies, in the light of comparisons with further cases. The theoretical bases of the method are explained in Appendix 1. For a fuller account of comparing and theorising from case studies, see Wengraf (2000, 2001), Rustin (1998b) and Cooper (2000).

Our argument in this book centres on a threefold typology: carers who are pulled into the home, those who are more outward-oriented, and those who are torn between the two spheres. From our 24 detailed case studies, we have chosen for presentation five or six from each society, two (where possible) for each subset of the typology. We have tried to maximise variety within as well as among societies.

Our purpose is not to generalise abstractly, but to use the case studies to illustrate key dynamics within each society, and as a basis for discussing carer situations and strategies and new approaches to social policy. We hope that readers will find the case studies numerous enough to give a rich and convincing feel for the dynamics and contexts we are describing, yet few enough to hold in mind. The cases presented are of course backed up in our minds by further detailed case studies and the other 60 or so interview profiles (see Appendix 2). The three cases outlined at the start of this chapter are also sometimes referred to.

The structure of the book

The book begins by introducing readers to the welfare context in each society and to particular carers. Much of the depiction of national and local welfare settings in West and East Germany and Britain in chapters two, three and four draws from interviews with local experts about the respective systems of community and domiciliary care. More detail is given in the case of East Germany, for which less background reading is available. Through this contextual knowledge we hope readers will be able to enter imaginatively into the life-worlds of the carers and consider the dynamics of informal systems of welfare in different societies, reflecting critically on the capacity of welfare systems to support people in meeting the challenges of caring in their lives.

The first three chapters aim to bring alive the 'Janus-headed' system (the term used by Leibfried and Ostner (1991)) of corporatism and subsidiarity in West Germany, the state socialist model of the former GDR, and the transition from social democratic collectivism to marketised liberalism in Britain. The chapters also relativise these terms, pointing to how the institutions they describe are embedded in and modified by wider social structures, including the informal sphere and civil society.

Chapter five focuses on the 'biographising' of caring. It explores differences in the significance of caring for individuals' lives, and between carers who can hold onto a sense of their past and future identities and those who become entrenched in the present. It discusses the way carers represent themselves, and the emphasis on agency in the case reconstruction approach to interpretation, using concepts of biographical or caring strategies. This contrasts with the passivity and social determinism which is implied in some life course approaches, and by the concept of trajectory. Chapter five also discusses the implications for support work of the biographical approach and of distinguishing different stages of the caring career. Context is to some extent set aside in this chapter, yet it re-emerges in asking which systems make which biographical patterns more likely, and which systems seem to offer help with 'biographising' or reflexive biographical work – or have more potential to do so.

Chapter six draws on the earlier chapters to show the crucial importance of informal social infrastructures in sustaining carers, helping them to maintain horizons beyond their initial caring situation. It discusses the seemingly paradoxical, even perverse, relationship between formal and informal systems in each society, and what this implies for a more cultural approach to social policy and welfare services. In West Germany, where subsidiarity's traditional encouragement of community and family and its more recent stress on self-help initiatives would lead one to expect a supportive communal life, carers seemed *least* likely to be drawn out of domestic isolation. East Germany, whose regime disavowed the very concept of civil society, gave rise to the most active informal engagement. And despite its voluntary tradition and relatively strong web of communal relationships, Britain seemed to lead carers, following energetic but eventually disappointing forays into the social world, to fall back on their own personal and family resources (Chamberlayne, 1999b, p 169). Understanding these paradoxes is of fundamental importance to the task of actively connecting social policy with everyday realities in a context of rapid social change. We compare the treatment of empowerment and the informal sphere in different social policy traditions, notably the Anglo-Saxon and the continental, and more recently in Third Way and European policy discourses.

Chapter Seven concludes with a discussion of caring as a political challenge. Here we summarise the significance of the study for emergent debates on citizenship and gender equality, as well as for a new cultural paradigm of social policy which emphasises biographical resources, cultural networks and personalised professional support.

Notes

[1] Our study pays some attention to, but does not specifically focus on, the perspective of the disabled person. In several cases, carees were present during the interviews, and sometimes participated.

[2] In this study we often use 'West German' synonymously with 'the Federal system', in order to distinguish from the East German system. The context should make it clear whether we are referring to the former geographical West German Federal area or the Federal system later covering the whole of Germany.

[3] Prue Chamberlayne heard of biographical-interpretive methods in March 1992 at the University of East London, during an ERASMUS exchange visit by Simone Kreher from Humboldt University. She tried out the method in pilot interviews in Leipzig during a 12-week research visit funded by the ESRC (on *Elderly people and neighbourhood networks*) in the summer of 1992. During that visit she and Annette King undertook training in the biographical-interpretive method, at Quatext in Berlin. The *Cultures of care* project began in November 1992, with Simone Kreher acting as methods consultant in Leipzig.

[4] The term socio-biographical method has somewhat superceded the terms 'hermeneutic biographical case reconstruction' and 'biographical-interpretive' method, used by us in previous publications (King and Chamberlayne, 1996; Chamberlayne and King, 1996). We sought a term which would emphasise our more contextualised use of biographical methods. Within the SOSTRIS project, the 'socio-biographical' method became the accepted terminology, at least within the British team (Chamberlayne and Rustin, 1999).

[5] The fact that the semi-structured pilot interviews were conducted in East Germany in the summer of 1992, while the restructuring of health and welfare services was still at a relatively early stage, was doubtless a strong reason for the peremptory nature of the responses. The questions focused on the interface with services, and it was unlikely that carers would give coherent and elaborated views of a system in a process of rapid change, about which they also had mixed feelings.

[6] Not all interviewees would respond to this open form of questioning, as is clear in several of the exchanges cited in Chapters Two to Four (see for example pp 70-1).

[7] Frauke Sinclair had an initial one-year appointment to work on the British part of the project, and in the uncertainty concerning the extension of her contract, got a job doing local authority research. Christine Jones worked half-time for a

year on the project. Susanne Rupp, who was experienced in the biographical method, was initially appointed for six months full-time, then transferred full-time for three years to the SOSTRIS project.

[8] Some life history methods tend to work more directly with the interviewee's subjective account in a process of giving voice; some are interested in the interviewer-effect, coproduction and power relations within the interview setting; some focus on collective representation and the social construction of accounts. For a fuller discussion of the diversity of narrative methods, see the introduction to Chamberlayne et al (eds) (2000).

TWO

West Germany – the pull into the home

Introduction

We begin the comparison of informal care in the three welfare societies, the two Germanies and Britain, with the West German case studies. We have chosen a similar structure for the first three chapters: a first section describes the context of the respective welfare society, through a discussion of salient themes of social policy and welfare praxis. A second section discusses the case studies, and in the final section of the chapter the cases are compared.

In this chapter on Western Germany, we argue that informal care is a contradictory arena, which bridges traditional and post-modern life courses. At the heart of the West German culture of care lies the social state tradition, in which gendered notions of private and public worlds continue to be perpetuated through conservative family legislation and welfare policies. Among the West German cases, most informal care was undertaken by women, with limited outside assistance and contact. This could be entrapping and restrictive, cutting carers off from outside contact and social interaction to the point of virtual isolation. For carers who managed to retain the connections to outside social spheres, acting against the grain of accepted social values, the experience of being a carer could become an arena for self-fulfilment, of experimentation in lifeworlds and a basis to reach out into new and unknown territory.

The social state tradition

In the corporatist model of the West German welfare state, social policy and social policy intervention are intrinsically linked with the tradition of the 'Sozialstaat' (Rosenhaft and Lee, 1997). Behind this lies the idea that the state can act as a mediator between changes and continuities of social life, between tradition and innovation in institutions and systems, and as a force for social cohesion (Peukert, 1990, p 345). Written into the Constitution, the aspiration of the social state is that of creating and maintaining a socially 'responsible' and progressive welfare society in which welfare functions are taken on by different sectors of society as a matter of social obligation and civil participation. Historically, the tradition of the social state continues the pluralist approach to welfare provision begun in the 19th century, in which welfare was developed as a civil endeavour, involving institutions such as unions, employers, churches and voluntary associations. These voluntary and civil institutions developed welfare services in the emerging industrial German state of the Wilhelmine Empire (Leibfried and Tennstedt, 1985). They became institutionalised as major providers of services in the Weimar Republic in the postwar period and produced a characteristic dual system of welfare provision, which combines state and independent welfare organisations under one institutional umbrella, balancing the requirements for strong civil, participatory society with those of coherent leadership through state policy. The relationship between state, family and intermediary welfare organisations is determined by the principle of 'subsidiarity'. Emerging out of the teachings of social Catholicism in the 19th century (Olk, 1986), subsidiarity enshrines an inverted hierarchy of welfare intervention, in which smaller units of society are given preference over larger units in taking on welfare responsibility: personal solutions to welfare risks are given precedence over collective, voluntary and state interventions. Within welfare policy, subsidiarity regulates the relationship between individuals and state, and safeguards the interests of smaller units, particularly the family, against the overpowering influence of the state. It supposedly taps into and at the same time perpetuates social interdependence, voluntarism, 'difference', and self-organisation.

After the disruption of Nazism, policy in the postwar period sought to regulate welfare intervention by retaining the plurality of strong autonomous providers in welfare, financed through the state. This policy approach was to encourage autonomous provision through self-help and individual and collective initiative, while guaranteeing the welfare of citizens through coordinated policy (Peukert, 1990; Leibfried and Ostner, 1991). It meant that the traditional occupation and church-based welfare organisations would be paid to provide welfare services, ranging from health advice centres to disability services, limiting the need for direct state or municipal welfare services.

Individual social welfare is comprehensively secured through a federally controlled, employment-centred social insurance policy, which provides comparatively generous payments and services, and is designed to compensate for risks of unemployment and for old age. In the breadwinner model of social security, benefits are focused on preserving the income and status of (male) wage earners, and paid as a proportion of previous earnings (Lewis and Ostner, 1992). For example, pension entitlements reflect the former earning power of employees; unemployment and sickness payments are also proportionate to earnings and are consequently more generous than flat-rate payments. This system was maintained even in the much tighter economic situation of the 1990s, despite the increasing fiscal burden (Ostner, 1993, p 92; also Peukert, 1990). In addition, transfer payments through tax breaks and family benefits are comparatively high in European terms.

This employment-based social insurance is complemented by a flat-rate social assistance system for welfare risks not covered through social insurance. In comparison to the benefits available through social insurance, social assistance has traditionally been less generous and is based on means-testing. While the social insurance system has remained largely unchanged, the scope and remit of social assistance administration has expanded over time to accommodate the changing realities of social need. As such, it has increasingly taken on the role of a welfare agency responsible for a growing diversity of clients. For example, the social assistance system administers claims for equipment for disabled people, as well as applications for various support services. For applicants, the cumbersome and long-winded nature of the application and assessment process, together with the time delays in receiving approvals, is a constant source of worry and annoyance.

In addition, the more volatile economic climate and labour market changes during the 1980s and 1990s have increased numbers from across the social spectrum who draw on social assistance at varying points in their lives, adding to the cost of the system. It is not surprising therefore that in recent years there have been increasing calls for a wholesale overhaul of the social security system to accommodate new 'welfare risks'. Social policy commentators such as Leisering and Leibfried (1999) call for a social security system that is sensitive to risks across the life course and can be responsive to a series of structural disadvantages. Policy makers are currently debating different options for reform of the social security system.

Family policies and the position of women

Family policies in West Germany have tended to actively promote the model of the traditional gendered family unit (Lewis and Ostner, 1992). They originated in the conservative social politics of the Federal Republic in the 1950s, when family policies were devised to maintain and protect the traditional family against the upheavals of the economic restructuring of the postwar period (Ostner, 1993). Policy during the formative period of the Federal Republic tended to institutionalise a gendered division of the private and public spheres, and supported a gender division in the home by subordinating women legally to their husbands. It favoured the male family breadwinner through the range of benefits and tax breaks, while family law treated mothers and children as dependants. For example, fathers were tested for social assistance entitlements, although mothers were assigned family responsibilities. The policies also penalised non-traditional families, and particularly single mothers, harshly. A particularly vicious piece of legislation was the federal housing policy during the 1950s and 1960s, which gave priority to families and at the same time allowed landlords to reject single mothers on 'moral' grounds, stigmatising them and their children even further.

Reforms in family laws and social legislation were made during the 1970s and 1980s. Today, the rights and needs of individual family members receive greater attention (Chamberlayne, 1990b). More recent developments include enhanced pensions rights for mothers and the upgrading of child benefit in 1997. There have also been important social changes concerning the family and the employment patterns of women. The number of married mothers who work increased from 38% in 1972 to 51.3% in 1994 (Althammer and Pfaff 1999, p 34). However, mothers appear to supplement family and household incomes through part-time work, rather than pursue independent careers. For example, in 1994, 27.5% of mothers with children between six and 14 worked under 20 hours a week, 13,3% worked 21-35 hours, and 20.2% worked full time. In Eastern Germany, despite high levels of unemployment, only 4.3% of mothers with children in this age group worked less than 20 hours per week, while 57.6% worked full-time (Althammer and Pfaff, 1999, p 34). This means that in Western Germany many married women with children still do not qualify for independent social insurance entitlements, especially pensions. The opportunity costs for qualified women is especially high: they lose out on the career advancement and higher income potential, widening the gap to their unmarried peers.

The family policies of the 1950s are noticeable in the life courses of the generation of the older female carers in our study. They all fit into the standardised biography of the housewife model. Very few of the women in the sample had independent careers when they were young, and most gave up work after they married and have been primarily homemakers ever since. The exceptions are those women from low-income households, for example Frau Jakob, one of the case studies in the next section, who have held low-paid jobs to supplement their husbands' income.

The traditional family unit of the working husband and the housewife mother remains a strong feature of West German society. The bias towards the traditional family unit in policy[1] has repercussions for the wider role of women, and the status of working mothers, non-traditional families and single parents, slowing down the impetus for change in attitudes to gender and family in the Federal Republic, and underpinning the continued gendered division of public and private spheres[2] (Ostner, 1993, p 96). These policies also create a division between traditional and non-traditional families, by privileging (heterosexual) coupledom and penalising other forms of arrangements. For example, the economic position of single mothers remains precarious: 50% of unmarried mothers live on incomes below the poverty line, and the majority of single working mothers earn comparatively little (Ostner, 1993; Klett-Davies, 1997)[3].

As in other European countries, the wider social position of women in West German society remains ambivalent. While the number of women entering higher education has risen dramatically in recent years and more married women have entered the labour market, occupational success and economic advancement lag behind their aspirations and life plans (Chamberlayne, 1994; Born and Krüger, 1993).

Attitudes towards the welfare society have remained broadly positive in that people in Germany still identify with the aims of welfare policies, if not necessarily with the increasing costs involved (Roller, 1992). Moreover, the life courses of the interviewees in West Germany broadly reflect the norms set by these policies. None of the younger women caring for children worked at all, and they did not expect to return to work soon. Women carried out most of the caring activities, while husbands, however supportive, were assistants rather than co-carers. In this sense, the 'Sozialstaat' idea has continued to be significant in personal ways as a normative framework of individual behaviour and identity. One might view this institutionalising of the life worlds of its citizens as continuing a form of 'social disciplining', in which welfare needs, aspirations and choices are moulded and through which social change is mediated and cushioned (Rosenhaft and Lee, 1997, p 27; Frevert, 1984; for the theory of social discipline see Foucault (1977) and Elias (1980)).

In our interviews with welfare representatives and carers, we found few challenges to the idea of a predominantly family-based system of informal caring. The overriding concern of the West German experts in the field, for example, was how to improve service provision for home-based care, and what additional services could be offered by the welfare organisations were care insurance to be established[4]. These debates centred on the fiscal consequences of care insurance, both for individuals and for the state. Similar viewpoints and worries were expressed in the interviews with carers. This was despite the fact that alternatives and independent forms of living are strongly promoted by representatives of disability organisations.

Politically, issues around family and gender were explicitly debated in the conservative initiative around 'new motherliness' in the early 1980s, which has attempted to valorise the work women do as mothers and to give equal social status to unpaid caring work. While rejected as an opportunist attack on women's labour market participation, left-wing and green politics have sought to develop their own models of validating informal and community reproductive work, resulting for example in a campaign for 'new subsidiarity' in the 1980s. This was to revive a greater self-reliance and self-help ethos in society, but has been viewed by many social commentators as a policy of welfare reduction rather than as a genuine attempt to harness people's self-help potential (Olk, 1986).

Among German feminists, the debate around 'new motherliness' has rekindled longstanding debates about the nature of femininity, and between 'difference' and 'equality' positions within feminism (Chamberlayne, 1990b). These debates critique simplistic equations between employment and emancipation. They point to the alienating effects of employment-based models of equality, which can produce their own set of dependencies, ethical problems and limitations for women. In practice, these debates have given rise to a number of different activities. A large number of women's projects experiment in forms of alternative living, attempting to find solutions beyond the narrow framework of 'work-home', 'housewife-mother' existence in the private sphere. In a study on single mothers, Mädje and Neusüss (1994) found that single women had developed increasing confidence and assertiveness in dealing with welfare authorities. They had come to view their welfare dependency as a rightful (but not necessarily adequate) compensation for their parenting efforts. While these discussions do not necessarily crystallise as welfare debates, they have been important as indicators of alternatives to traditional family life in Germany.

Service provision

The framework of benefits for disabled people and carers is part of the social assistance scheme, which includes a range of financial payments and services, financed through municipalities and the regional Länder. Of particular importance are schemes designed to assist people in special life circumstances (Hilfe in besonderen Lebenslagen, Hilfe zum Lebensunterhalt). Benefits available under these schemes are means-tested, but have high income thresholds and are therefore available to substantial groups of disabled people and also carers.

The organisation of personal social services is devolved to six welfare organisations, which play a major role in delivering services. These organisations are: the Arbeiterwohlfahrtsorganisation (AWO) (Workers' Welfare Organisation), Rotes Kreuz (Red Cross), Deutscher Paritätischer Wohlfahrtsverband (DPWV – umbrella association for independent smaller welfare organisations), Innere Mission (Protestant), Caritas (Catholic) and the Jewish Welfare Organisation (Lorenz, 1994; Clasen and Freeman, 1994). As professionally managed independent voluntary organisations, they maintain the specific characteristics of the membership constituency they have historically emerged from, and towards whom they are still allowed to a degree to target their services (Bauer, 1985).

While local and municipal authorities take on coordinating roles and provide capital funding, welfare organisations deliver services, such as domiciliary assistance and community nursing. In the city of Bremen, uniquely in Germany, the system of provision is geographically organised through a zoning of districts. This is different to the more common 'social station' (*Sozialstationen*) approach used in many areas, in that each welfare organisation is 'allocated' its share of territory in the city. From an administrative point of view, the system minimises the duplication of local service provision (and eliminates potential competition among welfare agencies) and anchors the welfare organisation within a specific locality. It also guarantees the geographical coverage of the whole of the city area. Service providers are based in neighbourhood centres, strategically located in the district. They are the local nerve centres for information and advice on services, and brokers for domiciliary care staff. Services provided range from nursing (often paid for through health insurance), domiciliary help and odd items such as transport or repair work. From the users' perspectives, the neighbourhood centres are well established within their localities and comprise a useful and, in many cases, quite personalised resource for local people, particularly older people.

Services are also provided through a range of other organisations, among them local churches, private providers, and disability and pressure groups who specialise in advice work and political lobbying. These last are mainly used by younger carers.

Provision for children and young people has remained as a principal arena of state regulation. Youth protection and youth development fall under the responsibility of regional Länder government as part of the Youth and Education Ministries. In Bremen, services for children and young people have a high political profile and extensive provision is available to children with disabilities. Services are sophisticated and progressive, and are conducted in conjunction with medical/hospital services and underpinned by a city-wide policy of integrated schooling for children with disabilities. There is little doubt that the specialised services for children, and the early treatment and support, are welcomed and highly esteemed by experts and parents alike. Once registered with the Bremen authorities as having special needs, children continue to receive services up to adulthood (18 years of age).

A number of the parents in our study had moved into the hinterlands of Bremen, but continued to take the option of participating in the early years support (*Frühförderung*), which provides a number of specialised and intensive developmental therapeutic services for (physically and learning) disabled children. When children switch to adult services, the young adults fall under the general service provision. For those experiencing the transition, provision can appear suddenly and dramatically reduced, and young people and their parents can feel abandoned, particularly when behavioural problems reduce options for day care.

Care insurance

During the 1970s and 1980s, the cost of care for dependent adults escalated, because of an increasingly older population without family support, as well as increasing costs of residential and nursing care which left many old people without the means to support themselves and dependent on social assistance. In turn, this led to crippling costs for the social assistance system. For those with sufficient personal means (or for their families), the cost of private residential and nursing care became prohibitively expensive. After protracted political negotiations, the solution adopted was to introduce in 1995 a compulsory, contributory care insurance on the lines of the health insurance system, securing financial and infrastructural benefits for those in need of care (Ruppel and King, 1995). This care insurance was the first major change in the insurance system since 1927.

Under the care insurance system, benefits based on care needs are available on the basis of medical and social assessment, but are capped (Kesselheim, 1999). While problems remain, care insurance has reduced some of the worries of the financial aspects of caring and dependency, and on the whole was highly welcomed by participants in the study[5].

The care insurance system was introduced in a climate of reduction in welfare state expenditure, in which health insurance and the institutions of social welfare were restructured with the explicit aim of cost savings (Ostner, 1998). For a time after its introduction, care insurance was used as a way for health insurance providers and social assistance boards to withdraw from participating in covering the costs of care in individual cases (Evers and Rauch, 1999). While such 'misunderstandings' of the financial complexities of individual cases were resolved eventually, this experience has raised a number of concerns about the corporate nature of social welfare in Germany under the tighter financial regimes. For commentators such as Kaufmann (1993), the introspection of state welfare agencies raises the question of whether the corporate approach to social welfare services is irrevocably damaged under the new fiscal managerial approach and administrative programme (Hermsen and Weber, 1998).

The introduction of care insurance sparked a proliferation of private and voluntary service providers who are competing for valuable contracts in this new industry of domiciliary and residential care. Some commentators welcome marketisation as increasing quality and choice of formal services in the community care sector (Landenberger, 1998). For others, marketisation undermines the role of the traditional welfare providers and demotes welfare organisations into subcontractors of state welfare. The concern among the established welfare organisations is that the current trend towards private payments interferes with the finely-tuned balance of the welfare system, and may endanger their existing expertise and commitment to client-centred approaches to service provision (Roth, 1999; Evers, 1997).

The West German cases

The 'pull into the home', characterising the West German cases, highlights the emphasis on family solutions in caring and the continued reliance on traditional gender roles. Characteristic of the West German cases is the tendency to 'resolve' the situation from within the informal sphere of the family, the home, and largely without outside help. Carers are often isolated in their situation, carrying the responsibility of care by themselves. The strategies are often internalised, if not at the beginning, but quite often during the process of care over time. Consequently, family-based care is difficult to sidestep. Carers who are faced with a caring challenge are easily drawn into the informal sphere of caring, devoting their time and life exclusively to this task. Links with public and social spheres diminish and the carer gets trapped in the informal sphere without opportunities to change the pattern of caring or gain outside support. The three typologies of carer strategies presented here show differentiation among these basic adaptation strategies in the West German cases.

Trapped in the private sphere

The cases in this category represent the most isolated caring set-ups: there is very little help, the situation is self-chosen, and the public and private spheres are quite separate; despite medically delicate situations there is little outside contact.

Both carers in this category are full-time. Frau Jakob's husband is highly dependent after a stroke, and she needs to attend to him most of the day and night. She has few outside contacts and even her family cannot or will not give her more support. She tolerates an increasingly isolated life until her husband's death. Frau Hamann adopts a similarly isolating caring strategy. Although she has a professional qualification and career, she takes on her son's nursing role on a full-time basis, with little family or professional support. In her case, caring implies giving up a thriving medical career for her family and increasing dependence on her husband.

Frau Jakob

> Herr Jakob has been in a wheelchair since a stroke in 1989. He has a further
> stroke in 1991, which paralyses him. He is bed-bound and dependent on
> tubular feeding, and requires 24-hour care. Frau Jakob, 59, takes him home
> against medical advice. Herr Jakob needs complex nursing interventions;
> Frau Jakob has learned how to do them and carries out most of the caring
> work herself. She is assisted by a nurse for 23 hours a week, a service which
> she partly has to pay for herself. In addition to these hours, she occasionally
> has a Zivi, who will carry out errands for her or sit with her husband while
> she goes out.

Frau Jakob works part-time as a cleaner in a GP's surgery early in the
morning – her husband is left alone for this period. Socially, she has few
contacts apart from her sisters and her son and his family. She tends to
keep a distance from neighbours and expects little in terms of support,
although she is very willing to help others out. It is a punishing schedule
of round-the-clock caring, with very few and rushed breaks and an
increasingly isolated existence. Frau Jakob herself sums up her complete
commitment to caring as a life motto at the beginning of the second
interview: "if at all, then properly".

Frau Jakob was born in the 1930s. She comes from a working-class
family; her mother works as a shop assistant and her father is a sailor. The
family set-up is a traditional one where daughters are raised in
housekeeping skills. The girls learn 'out of house' in domestic employment.
Frau Jakob talks with some pride of the professional training she has
received in a dentist's household from the age of 16, first as an apprentice
for three years and then in domestic service. She marries in 1959 and has
a son in the early 1960s. Frau Jakob talks very little about her married
life; her life revolves around her child and her own family. Outside social
contacts are limited to her husband's work colleagues.

In the early 1980s, her father falls ill suddenly and dies in hospital from
an undiagnosed cancer.

Interviewer:	Would you have cared for your parents, if it had come to that?
Frau Jakob:	Yes, yes. We did, my sister and I. Everybody went .... We drove there anyway, but when she was alone, one week I went, shopping and so forth.... The other week

> my sister went, then the youngest, she did the washing. And Sunday and Saturday, the grandchildren went, the brother-in-laws. My mother wanted to stay alone. And so we went.... She wouldn't have come.

Interviewer: Did your mother care for your father?

Frau Jakob: No, my father went to hospital on Sunday or Monday, and Tuesday he passed away. And my mother felt guilty that he passed away because she took him to hospital. If she had kept him at home.... So he passed away, very quietly. And my mother passed away at home. On Thursday, I went there and my brother-in-law, we met and everything was tidy, and Saturday the neighbour rang, when the curtains were open and the milk still stood in front of the door. And so the neighbour rang my youngest sister. My sister went there and she [the mother] had passed away. She passed away Friday to Saturday, because we – we had been there on Thursday. It was like that.

This idealised account of 'family-centred' care for her parents is in marked contrast to her actual caring experiences with her husband. Herr Jakob's illness is long and undignified in its consequences. After his second stroke, he is offered a residential nursing care bed. Frau Jakob rejects this, because she feels compelled to carry on with her role as carer. The care regime is tiring and difficult and takes over her life. Caring increasingly isolates her: dismayed at her decision to care at home, her family does not offer much assistance and she herself has never learned to involve outside agencies in her 'private' family realm. Herr Jakob dies in 1993, a short time before the second interview. After his death, Frau Jakob's life does not change significantly. Embittered and drained by the years of caring, she remains isolated and lonely.

Frau Jakob's ideas about a satisfying and appropriate caring situation remain unfulfilled. She misses the close network of family relations, the sharing of caring and domestic tasks with other family members and the emotional bonds that go with it – all of which had been part of caring for her parents. An important factor in her decision to care at home is her intransigent stance of what she 'ought' to do in this particular situation. Frau Jakob draws on traditional normative ideas about (female) family duty and responsibility, about serving family needs, and a pride in appropriate domestic management, about (self-)limitation of individual ambitions and choices, and about loyalty to family members. She has carried this identity forward, but in relation to her life as a carer it has impoverished her socially and emotionally. She is dependent on the informal sphere, without receiving reciprocal attention. Frau Jakob is unwilling to and incapable of adjusting to changing circumstances and has a limited repertoire of alternative courses of action to make her life more bearable. Consequently, her frustrations are directed towards her family, which has let her down by not responding in providing the extensive family support she wishes for.

Frau Hamann

Frau Hamann is 34. Her two-year-old son, Matte, has serious developmental problems, which are the consequence of a non-specific neurological disorder. He is also physically quite fragile. The family have a younger son, Kai, who is ten months old. Frau Hamann is a neurologist, specialising in paediatrics. She undertakes Matte's nursing and medical care.

Until 1990, Frau Hamann has been training for a promising medical career in neuro-paediatrics in a university hospital in Southern Germany. She meets her future husband on a skiing holiday. After four months of heart-searching she leaves her partner of nine years' standing and her career, and moves north to be with her new love. At that time her future husband is still married. She works temporarily in a local paediatric surgery and then as a dental assistant and surgery manager in her new partner's dental surgery, until her son is born. Her new family situation is complicated and insecure, with acute hostility from her prospective in-laws, who own the dental practice and have withdrawn support from the family. Her own family disapproves of her giving up her promising career in medical research. Matte is seven months old when the couple marry.

After marriage, her situation does not improve. She has had few opportunities to make new friends and her social life is limited. The children require constant attention and her husband is preoccupied with work and financial problems. Frau Hamann feels very isolated; her only regular contact is with the child developmental worker, who works with Matte on a regular basis. Frau Hamann's isolation is compounded by a lack of understanding from her husband. He anticipates that she will assist him again in the surgery and she foresees great battles if she decides to resume work as a medical doctor rather than as her husband's assistant.

Frau Hamann experiences her situation as confusing and deeply traumatic, as 'suffering' – in biblical tones – and not life. She is torn between her independent identity as professional and doctor, and her dependency as mother, wife and carer in the home. For her, the two roles are incompatible; at the same time, both constitute axes for her subjective fulfilment as a person. In the interview structure this is reflected in the constant change in perspective between 'me as doctor' and 'me as mother/wife', and the consistent reflexivity in the account and (academic) disputation with the interviewer:

> As soon as Matte was born, I knew, I myself as mother, immediately actually, that something was wrong. I knew because I am myself a doctor, by chance or by fate. I worked in neuro-surgery and therefore couldn't misinterpret the symptoms.

Nevertheless, when her son is first born, she ignores the symptoms for some time. She goes home as the happy mother, until her son becomes seriously sick and she can no longer deny that he has problems.

Her son's incipient disability and the need to draw on her professional background to care for him has shattered the dream of the family life she had striven for. Reflecting on her situation as 'fate' is Frau Hamann's only way of articulating her unhappiness and the anger she experiences at her designated role as 'professional carer in the private sphere'. At present, her husband and the family are beyond recourse – whether they will remain so intransigent is a different matter. With greater experience in her situation and the growing wish to move on, she may be able to develop the personal and objective resources to undertake different courses of action.

On one level, Frau Hamann's life trajectory represents the traditional female move into the housewife model after marriage. On another, the traumatic circumstance of the transition, the break-up of her longstanding relationship, her arrival as the 'other woman' and the birth of her child before marriage contain an element of going against the norms, signified in the disapproval of her elders' generation. In her commitment to the new relationship she has cut herself off from her previous life, leaving professional status and development, informal networks and family behind. What provides some status is her medical work in relation to her son. Yet his condition is not operable and in that sense not medically treatable, leaving her expertise largely untapped.

Painful compromises

The two cases in this category continue the theme of the dilemma many West German women face in combining caring responsibilities with a life outside the home. Like Frau Hamann, Frau Hegemann and Frau Luchtig both have great difficulties in carrying out their caring duties and maintaining outside interests. Frau Hegemann cares for her husband and is committed to a full family life. She is also the breadwinner and manages a household single-handedly. This is an exhausting existence and not very rewarding. Similarly, Frau Luchtig cares for her mother and manages to maintain a full artistic career. The experience of both women is that the pull into the informal sphere of caring is always stronger than the other activities or plans. The pockets of independent living are continuously under threat either through changing circumstances of illness or disability, or through the tensions in the home deriving from the caring situation.

Through their continuing negotiation efforts, they manage to maintain caring at home and in both cases also maintain an outside life. This is a personally costly process and includes difficult family relationships, but has meant that they have not become as entrapped and isolated as Frau Jakob and Frau Hamann.

Frau Hegemann

Herr Hegemann is diagnosed with multiple sclerosis (MS) in 1980 at the age of 30, cutting short an army career. His condition has deteriorated substantially over the years so that today he hardly ever goes downstairs or out of the house. Additionally, he suffers from a very painful kidney condition. He is cared for mainly by his wife, but, following a hospital stay, a nurse comes in during the week for Herr Hegemann's personal care for two hours each morning. Frau Hegemann now insists on this additional help. Herr Hegemann remains on his own during the day until his wife or his children come back in the afternoon.

The Hegemanns have three children: two sons, aged 24 and 21, and a 13-year-old daughter. All the children continue to live at home. The children have their duties but, according to Frau Hegemann, they do not help a lot. She still services them, to the dismay of her husband.

Frau Hegemann is the breadwinner of the family since her husband's pension is not sufficient to support them. She works full-time in a bank, a job she enjoys. She feels she gets the necessary intellectual stimulation and company at work in a friendly, all-female working team. In the early years after the diagnosis of the illness, the couple switch domestic roles, with Herr Hegemann looking after the youngest daughter as a househusband.

At the beginning of the interview, Frau Hegemann remarks that their approach to the illness has always been to 'grow' with the situation. She rejects the idea that her situation is unusual enough to be 'worth' a story:

> And therefore we didn't have many problems in the beginning. *For none of us.* In the first instance, we never worried about what will be tomorrow. [six-second pause] We don't even do that today very much.

In response to developing the physical symptoms of MS at the age of 30, the family devise a number of daily rituals over the years, in an attempt to circumvent Herr Hegemann's increasing lack of mobility and physical limitation. An example of this is the ritual of afternoon tea, which is taken in Herr Hegemann's room after Frau Hegemann's return from work. In this way, the family integrates Herr Hegemann's illness into the normal routine of family life, a strategy that works well for many years.

In recent years, the situation has become more difficult and strains show in the family. Herr Hegemann's ability to participate in family life diminishes due to the progress of the illness. He reacts by becoming increasingly authoritarian. The Hegemanns' teenage daughter has serious clashes with her father. As her husband's life is restricted to his room, Frau Hegemann becomes his mouthpiece, drawing her into conflicts and forcing her to take 'sides'. On one occasion the oldest son is excluded from the family home, at quite a young age. He eventually returns, but the tensions in the home are growing and the gulf between the parents and children is widening. Frau Hegemann realises her impossible position at the centre of these different factions and interests in her family. Nevertheless, she remains loyal to her husband, alienating the children in the process.

The Hegemanns have become isolated from their formerly thriving networks of friends and acquaintances; and they are largely without other informal support. Herr Hegemann's only phone contact is with his sister.

Frau Hegemann's contact with her own family is sporadic. The increased demands on her time and energy at home also affect the relative independence her working life used to offer her. She has less opportunity to go out with her work colleagues, and her enjoyment of work is marred by feelings of guilt about her relative independence, compared with her husband's increasing dependency.

Although problems are mounting, for many years the family has done well in living with their strategy of normalising the illness. As a result, the couple have maintained a strong marital partnership and they can offer each other mutual support. It has made them an 'example of excellence' in the eyes of the MS group:

> Frau Hegemann: We were always portrayed as the example.
>
> Interviewer: Why? Because you have such a long experience?
>
> Frau Hegemann: No, not because we had it a long time, but because we dealt differently with the situation than others, because we didn't go mad with worry, didn't look up everything, in order to know what to expect. We didn't burden ourselves with difficult future prospects, but we tried to carry on living as before. And we lived well ... on the whole.

Being presented as exemplary also gives the couple status and prestige in the MS circle, which for some years might have been a positive experience. However, over the years, living with this label seems to have turned into a burden of expectation. It has possibly contributed to reducing social contacts, because the effort of living up to this external expectation of 'normality' might be too difficult to fulfil: watching the losing battle of physical decline of somebody who was supposed to be 'coping' well, as well as stresses and strains in the family members is something they wanted to keep private.

The problem for the Hegemanns is the inertia and routine in day-to-day living, which dominates the normalisation strategy and does not allow for development. The Hegemanns do not take the changing context of the illness (increasing dependency) and the transformation of relationships within the family unit (children reaching adulthood) into account. They remain marooned in a family dynamic which has turned the household into a battle zone between parents and children. This stagnation in family relationships keeps all family members from moving on in their lives. The children cannot gain the independence of adult life by remaining in the house, and the parents cannot plan for the future:

> [laughs] We dream that the children are grown up and move out and we get a nice small three-room apartment on the ground floor.

Frau Luchtig

> Frau Luchtig has a longstanding career as a family carer: all her life she has looked after her parents and now cares for her mother, who is in her eighties and frail. Frau Luchtig regards her caring activities as dominating her whole life. Frau and Herr Luchtig have shared a house with her parents, she has worked in the family business – a shop – and today her mother lives in a small flat above her. The mother is ailing, although still mobile and otherwise independent. Financially, she derives income from her daughter for the flat and from the lease of her shop. They also have a cleaner, and somebody goes for walks with her mother twice a week.

Frau Luchtig is born into a lower middle-class family during the war. From a young age, she has to work in the shop in her spare time, or look after her younger brothers. She does well at school and is encouraged by her teachers. Her parents are not interested in her education and she leaves school at 15 to work for her parents in the shop. By contrast, her brothers finish school and obtain professional qualifications. In a bid for independence, her sister enters a convent and qualifies as a nurse.

> I came to work in the shop very early on, I was put into it, homework no, school, that was never important for my parents, studying. I would have loved to study music and art, but I could only do that later privately, it wasn't possible. And this is how it was.

Frau Luchtig is the only child who stays at home. She marries at 17, has a son, and the family continues to live with her parents. A few years into the marriage, the Luchtigs are able to afford to set up independently, but Frau Luchtig cannot leave her parents' control and so they remain tenants in her parents' home. They have spent all their married lives in close proximity to her parents, who even accompany them regularly to the weekend house.

Frau Luchtig resents this lack of privacy and her parents' interference with her adult life, but has been unable to change it. When her father dies in the 1980s, the chances for a more independent life become even more remote. There is not much love lost between Frau Luchtig and her mother. As the mother gets older and more dependent on her daughter, the power relations change and the mother becomes increasingly dependent on her daughter's contacts and efforts to entertain her.

> Well, I wouldn't advise it. We have a son, and I don't know, whether parents, whether they cannot separate from their children, if they are always together in the house. She is so demanding and doesn't seem to notice.

> How did I cope? I had a time when it was really awful. I said, this cannot be true. I said, let's move out, let's get away from here. So that we can be by ourselves for a bit. It didn't work.

In compensation for her lack of career, Frau Luchtig develops a variety of hobbies. While she has never received a formal artistic education, she has taught herself to play an instrument and skills in sculpturing and other artistic techniques:

> So I found some hobbies and played a lot of music [one second pause] co-founded an orchestra and we played a lot of music and other things, and the dolls. Ceramic dolls, painting courses. And this compensated a bit. You just have to build up something like that, otherwise you can't cope. I never trained for a career. The parents said, why do you need a career, you are at home and manage the shop. I worked as a sales assistant after we sold the business, when Marcus turned six.... After that, I was only at home here with my parents, always at hand and my husband didn't want to.

Over time, she turns her 'private' hobbies into professional activities, which become a considerable source of earnings and local recognition. She plays an important role in managing and conducting the local orchestra, and her artisan work is regularly exhibited in craft fairs.

Frau Luchtig can draw on her existing local network of friends and acquaintances to organise company and support in looking after her mother. By inviting friends to her house to spend time in her mother's company, she frees afternoons and evenings to do her 'own' thing. She skilfully dresses up these sitting services as 'entertainment sessions' to circumvent her mother's resistance to outside help:

> I invite friends and acquaintances to my house quite often. They spend an enjoyable few hours together in conversation. This is interesting for my mother, who will sit with them. In the meantime, I can go out to do what I need to. My friends don't mind, they know the situation here.

As a coping strategy for balancing her own interests and aspirations within a framework of family restriction and powerlessness in relation to her parents, Frau Luchtig has managed an ingenious solution to protecting her own sphere and negotiating the caring responsibilities around it, working around her mother's attempts at controlling her daughter's life.

Nevertheless, the hard fought-for freedom is threatened by potential developments in the future. If her mother, for example, should become frailer, Frau Luchtig's extensive social life and professional existence as an artist will once more be threatened. Also, there is the possibility that her husband will increase his demands on her time once he retires. Frau Luchtig feels anxious and threatened:

> I don't know what happens with my caring. If she becomes bedridden, I am fixed to the house. I'll try to work at home, I don't know what will happen to me.... Then there is my fear about my husband, with his heart attack. He recovered well, but I could have another caring case in the house. It all went well, but....

Frau Luchtig is adamant that she could not give up caring for her mother or any other family member, that in the end she will have to sacrifice her artistic career to fulfil her obligation as a daughter or wife. But while Frau Luchtig's assessment of her future is rather bleak, her past ingenuity might help her to find a solution for the future.

Working the system

While the previous two cases constructed difficult compromises in their personal lives to accommodate caring, the two carers in this category have more decisively broken with the traditional boundaries between public and private worlds. They have developed a proactive relationship with the formal support services. Frau Mahler uses her social work background in developing a caring strategy for her foster daughter which is beneficial to her personally, to the financial security of her family, and for her foster daughter. Frau Alexander starts out dependent on the medical profession to look after her seriously sick son, but with time is able to break with this dependency and devise her own way of caring for him. Through this experience she becomes an assertive fighter for his welfare and is able to develop a rewarding life for him and the whole family. While Frau Mahler transcends the boundaries of family and professionalism, Frau Alexander has to rebuild the boundaries of a family life from a situation of hospitalisation.

Frau Mahler

Frau Mahler is 31 and cares for a disabled foster daughter, aged five. She has two other children, aged 11 and three. At the time of the second interview she is expecting a further child. Stella, her foster child, comes into the family at the age of 18 months as an emergency placement. Stella has Down's syndrome. In her foster family, she adjusts quickly and makes considerable developmental progress. The family decide to foster her long-term.

The Mahlers have only recently settled in a rather remote village outside Bremen. Here they are living with Herr Mahler's grandmother, who can no longer live alone and requires some degree of assistance. The family regards the current living arrangement as reciprocal, solving problems for both parties.

Herr Mahler is in the process of completing his nautical studies, which will enable him to work in merchant shipping as a senior officer or a captain. In the meantime, he works in a residential home for adults with disabilities. Frau Mahler is a qualified social worker and has worked with disabled children in the past. She has been approached by the youth service to consider fostering. The couple are experienced in looking after children with disabilities. Frau Mahler's professional qualifications enable her to come to a specific set of administrative arrangements with the youth service.

The Mahlers' decision to foster is a spontaneous one. Frau Mahler is pregnant with her second child at the time. She has had a number of miscarriages before, and it is her husband who suggests that having a baby in the house might distract Frau Mahler from brooding over her pregnancy. So they decide to take Stella on a short-term basis:

43

> Well it was really quite sudden. They phoned us a few times, wanted to see the flat – we never had a chance to send off the paperwork; I was special because I had worked for the youth service. They phoned on the Wednesday, whether we wanted Stella, ... and we had her on Thursday at eleven.

The arrangement is an immediate success and Stella makes her mark on the family very quickly:

> Well she came in through the door, Stella saw me, opened her arms and landed on my lap – and didn't want to leave it. The mother went after an hour and this is how we came to our daughter. [laughs]

> After two weeks ... even at that time, nobody could imagine, from the outside, that she had not always lived with us. I have never seen this in the whole of my professional life, nor has her social worker or the people from the early development section.

While Stella's mother remains in contact for around two years, eventually she gives up Stella for adoption and severs all contact. For financial reasons, the Mahlers decide not to adopt Stella, but negotiate quasi-adoptive rights over her, and are closely involved in the decision making about Stella's welfare. Frau Mahler is given the professional responsibility to monitor and further Stella's development herself. She can draw on the help of the youth service at any time. The Mahlers also have guarantees that Stella will not be taken away from them. The core of the arrangement is the continued financial help they receive from the youth service – fees and supplements they would lose if they decide to adopt. These financial benefits present a substantial income for this student household.

The Mahlers, because of their professional backgrounds, are well placed to benefit from the system of services. They can do so by assuming control over their own relationship to the services. Frau Mahler has no problems in transcending her roles as Stella's mother and professional social worker, of breaking down the boundaries of the public and private worlds for the benefit of the family. She integrates her professionalism as a social worker and educationalist with her own wish for a varied and extended family life. Central to this is the support of her husband in negotiating the technical details of the arrangements. She manages her daily life with the help of her considerable network of friends and also her mother, who moves in for a while to help out.

For Frau Mahler, the traditional privacy of conventional family and the public sphere are not incompatible — she and her husband transcend this divide. Significant are the emotional benefits the arrangement has brought. Frau Mahler thinks that Stella's original placement was instrumental for the survival of her new child. Through the diversion which Stella brought at a critical point in her pregnancy, she was able to stretch her pregnancy to term. Frau Mahler is expecting yet another child and might in the future want to foster a further child. The family has plans to live with friends and their children in the extensive new house they are planning to build.

Frau Alexander

> Frau Alexander has an 11-year-old child, Andre, who has a congenital heart and lung defect, which makes his breathing erratic and feeding difficult. He needs constant supervision, particularly at night. Frau Alexander has cared for him at home since they had him discharged from hospital at the age of two. He is tube-fed and has undergone numerous operations. The Alexanders have a second child, Sophie, who is seven.

Herr and Frau Alexander are in their mid-30s. Both come from a similar lower middle-class background. After leaving school, Frau Alexander starts a clerical job, for which she has little interest. Her husband is a master craftsman. There are few indications that the couple have any specific aspirations for their family; they expect to lead an ordinary family life. Their social network is centred on a local motorcycle club, to which the family has belonged for a long time. They attend biker meetings on a regular basis and spend much of their leisure time touring with the group.

Andre is born with a variety of congenital problems and initially is not expected to survive. He is in a hospital which is three hours' drive away across the river. Frau Alexander initially visits him only three to four times a week, but eventually spends all day in the hospital, taking over his nursing care. Although she is shy and intimidated by the surroundings, she begins to assert herself in the medical environment and starts to make more independent decisions about her son's care.

> One was too inexperienced then and one had a child and the child was disabled, one didn't know anything other than the hospital and what a doctor says is good and true and somehow one goes by that.

Because of his medical problems, the Alexanders are advised not to care for Andre at home. After a draining two years of travelling to and from the hospital and with increasing signs of institutionalisation in their child, the couple decide to take their son home, against medical advice. For the first period at home, Frau Alexander experiences great personal difficulties in managing her son's care, and receives very limited nursing input. She only survives by taking prescribed tranquillisers. Then there is a turning point for the family. They regain control over their family life and set out to forge it according to their own ideas.

> It took about a year, until I got used to it. I had to take drugs because I couldn't stand it, I was always in the twilight. I wanted to manage it, somehow I had to manage it for myself, but somehow I was all to pieces, but even so, you've got to do it. That lasted about three months. But then it went all fine, on his side there weren't actually any more problems.

Through her dedicated care, Andre's condition exceeds the highest expectation of his survival and development. Surviving those difficult three months shapes Frau Alexander's determination to fight for the very best for her child. Over the years, she asks for and receives a lot of help. Initially, a nurse comes for three hours a day, and Frau Alexander is allocated a home physiotherapist. She has a designated nurse in the kindergarten which Andre attends. Today, a nurse accompanies him to and from school and he receives occupational therapy on a regular basis.

Frau Alexander is cynical and critical of the competences of the medical profession. She is quite prepared to challenge medical advice and has in the past delayed operations and other medical intervention. Growing in confidence in their own abilities, the Alexanders have a second child when Andre is six. They build their own home, in part financed through the cash benefits they receive, and made a reality by Herr Alexander's do-it-yourself. They buy a camper van, which gives them much greater flexibility and mobility and allows them to take part in biker events. Surviving and succeeding in caring for Andre has given the family a sense of purpose, and great ingenuity and efficiency in managing their affairs. They have become a formidable 'team'. Apart from their connection to the biker community, the family is conventional. Frau Alexander takes care of the family and leaves employment to her husband. She has no intention of returning to work. They have no family support system to fall back on, and the support of friends is limited, since they are dispersed. Apart from formal services in the home and at school, Frau Alexander does not receive much help.

Perhaps because her coping strategy has been to resolve problems within a narrowly defined private environment, Frau Alexander finds it difficult to relate to the culture of carer and self-help groups, which rely on sharing experiences and learning from each other. It may also be that such groups cannot tackle deeper emotional issues either, and that Frau Alexander feels frustrated by that fact:

> One had the impression with a lot of people who were there that they were also very desperate, partly, with one mother, she was also full of problems and these problems certainly haven't gone away or anything, but ... it's a shame somehow.

Frau Alexander's self-sufficiency has its costs. She has never allowed herself to address the emotional trauma of the early years, and as Andre grows up and the situation settles down, she finds it difficult to develop a more ordinary 'parental' relationship with him:

> It was amazing, last year, when Andre went on a four-day class trip, well it was quite ridiculous. I didn't know what to do with myself here, this calm, the emptiness somehow.

She has never had the time to address the trauma of having a severely disabled child. She cannot express such feelings directly, but they lurk behind the practical issues she has been mainly preoccupied with:

> Your whole life, with this disabled child you have somehow changed your whole life, you've adapted to the situation, you've had to change your whole way of life, and that costs a lot of money.

The issue of sharing and receiving wider social support, including on emotional matters, is increasing in importance because her son now has substantial behavioural problems with which she has difficulty dealing. As this is unlikely to be solved through practical solutions, Frau Alexander may find it increasingly difficult to address the changing care needs of her son adequately.

Comparisons

A first comment on these case studies has to be that the gender and family roles, which structure informal family care, largely follow traditional family lines. Women are drawn into caring by virtue of their status as daughters, wives and mothers. The older carers especially conform to the gendered role of carer in the private sphere and have accepted this as a lifetime occupation. For some, caring is an extension of their previous housewife lives and aspirations, such as in the cases of Frau Jakob or Frau Alexander. It is also characteristic that women take on the caring role alone, without active support through partners or through family or friends.

The case studies illustrate the mobilising of personal circumstances and resources to meet the challenge of caring. The Mahlers operate within a professional field of childcare and pedagogy to create a framework for caring for their foster daughter, which allows them to use the system in a very particular way. West German caring cases echo British theorising about reciprocity and obligation in family relations, and the interplay of emotional and material dimensions in moulding modern intra-family relations and exchanges (Lewis and Meredith, 1988; Finch and Mason 1993, Ungerson; 1987). Finch (1989) has suggested a model of reciprocity in families which both accommodates and expresses social change. Monolithic norms have given way to a more individually differentiated pattern and rather finely tuned understandings of what constitutes obligations and who ought to care. While structural elements such as class and family roles still come into play, there is a sense in which these have been transcended and have given way to more individualised interpretations, allowing a diversity of formulations in deciding 'the right thing to do'.

Within the West German context, however, the strong normative framework guiding caring decisions remains pervasive in the home-orientedness of caring, 'pulling' informal carers into the private world of the home and family. The fluidity of values and negotiated patterns of care occur from within the private context of care, rather than challenging it. Developments and variations among West German carers seem to occur against the backcloth of the normative framework of family, normative gender roles, and a service structure which is geared towards servicing the informal sphere, rather than intervening in it.

Caring in the traditional family

In the cases discussed above, there is an undercurrent of an 'either–or' dichotomy in caring decisions, particularly in relation to combining family and employment. There is a very strong normative pull for women to enter an exclusive caring career. Frau Hegemann, for example, enjoys her job. At the same time, she feels ambivalent about it. She keeps it subordinated to her caring duties, but also quite hidden and separate from her family life. Another case, not discussed in detail in this book, is Frau Igel, who cares for her mother. She marries late and does not have any children of her own. When her mother starts to suffer from dementia, she gives up her job to care for her, despite the fact that her father is the main carer and there are constant tensions between father and daughter. Frau Igel cannot imagine not caring for her mother: "She is my mum, what else am I supposed to do?".

The conflict between normative roles and actual lifestyles is fought out as a daily dilemma for women such as Frau Hamann, who has a foothold in 'both' worlds. Part of her motivation in getting married and in giving up her career is that she embraces an identity as mother and carer. She seems to accept isolation as part of the meaning of mothering and caring. Frau Luchtig's inability to defy her mother's demands indicates the pervasive hold of the carer role; her other roles remain subordinated to her caring identity.

One way of overcoming the dilemma between personal aspirations and traditional gender roles, between the private family sphere and employment or external activity, is by becoming an 'outsider' to the traditional family setting. Here, developing a carer identity can be a more positive and enriching experience. The Alexanders (who themselves do not come from strong traditional family backgrounds) use caring as a springboard for enriching developments, while maintaining a close and in part traditional family set-up. This is also true for the Mahler family, who do not conform to the breadwinner ideal of the family setting. Actively supported by her husband, Frau Mahler's professional connections enable her to achieve financial security and develop a social arena of communal and open family life, in which boundaries of public and private are no longer counterposed.

Overall, the framework for informal caring in West Germany continues and sometimes reinforces traditional family patterns and gender role divisions between the private and public spheres. Despite feelings of resentment and emotional upheaval, there is little questioning in the interviews about alternatives. Carers might find the experience difficult and paralysing, but even in the most traumatic circumstances they cannot imagine a fundamentally different setting to caring.

Responding to change

A breakdown in family relations is one common source of crisis. Frau Luchtig's mother does not express any gratitude or feeling towards her daughter. This creates an emotional vacuum for Frau Luchtig as her labour of love is not returned, turning her effort into exploitation. The resulting emotional damage is significant.

Frau Hamann's case can also be seen as a breakdown in the reciprocal exchanges and relational obligations within family life. Frau Hamann is isolated and rejected within her married family, and her husband is unwilling or unable to compensate. As a consequence, Frau Hamann is denied the personal fulfilment in a caring role that she clearly craves and which she has not received within her professional career. Frau Jakob similarly falls foul of the shortcomings of other family members (her incapacitated husband, her sisters, her brother-in-law, her son), who do not keep their side of the bargain. Frau Hegemann's problem is slightly different: while she still fulfils the role of carer, she cannot keep up her other obligations. She cannot give her children the attention they want, and has increasing problems with them. Her situation is further complicated by her husband's deterioration, which makes it impossible to keep up with the conflicting demands. Caring in this way is an exhausting strategy and if the reciprocal family support networks are not functioning, the caring experience becomes oppressive and entrapping. The fragile arrangements that keep the situation under control dissipate. Little additional support can be drawn in and caring becomes an isolating and isolated activity.

The cases also show that crises are not an inevitable outcome of the traditional home-oriented caring paths. Frau Alexander, Frau Mahler and to some degree Frau Luchtig, all very much carers in their own home, have been very successful in controlling the demands on them for caring, and in developing resources for themselves and their families. Frau Alexander is a skilled negotiator with public authorities, Frau Mahler has a well-functioning private and public support system and Frau Luchtig organises her acquaintances to cover for her. Operating from within the private family sphere, these women have created caring strategies that reach outside the private realm of the family to gather strategic support and assistance. They thereby not only protect the family interests, but develop other aspects of their own skills and competences.

The ingredients of reciprocity, obligation and public identity carry carers culturally through difficult times. Frau Mahler uses her professional background as an educational social worker to maintain some distance from the demands of her own situation and to mobilise help for longer-term and shorter-term plans, such as the house building and saving plans for the children. In helping out an organisation in crisis, she can draw on increased attention and support for her whole family. In Frau Alexander's case, by her risky and dramatic decision to take her son home, and by improving his health and quality of life, she has been able to build up a great deal of professional credibility, which allows her to strive for improvements and services which benefit not only her son, but the whole family.

Services

Within the German social assistance framework, most of the services and advice available are organised into the home. This can be very convenient logistically, for instance for families with children. However, for Frau Hamann, it increases her isolation, because she does not have many other opportunities to socialise. Also, Frau Luchtig's most dearly held wish, that her mother should develop a social life of her own to make her more independent, is not furthered by the fact that the services would come into the house, an intrusion her mother rejects. It inhibits socialising and reinforces isolationist tendencies within home caring. For Frau Luchtig, service arrangements which would actively take her mother outside the home and be less obviously related to relieving her input as carer might be a more acceptable solution to her mother.

There is little evidence that the different welfare organisations involved with the various carers could address these issues within the scope of the services they were offering. Services were fairly homogeneous in the different districts, and while the staff in the neighbourhood centres were sympathetic to the needs of their carer clients and vulnerable people, individual differences could only be met in a very limited way. The 'care packages' available to children were much more tailored to individual situations, although parents' own needs could only be marginally considered. Frau Alexander's extensive nursing support in the early years of Andre's life was a major concession to her.

Although services and financial support are generous, they are not necessarily available immediately. Frau Mahler, Frau Alexander and Frau Hamann are entitled to extensive children's and educational services, but securing them is still an elaborate bureaucratic process. Both Frau Hamann and Frau Mahler, because of their professional connections, have found this process relatively uncomplicated. Frau Alexander, however, has had to fight every inch of the way, beginning with the release of her son from hospital. However, she has learned a great deal and is now able to take on the complex bureaucracy in fighting for disability benefits for her son.

Among the older carers, the situation is more complex. Frau Jakob receives community nursing care, but very little else in terms of services. This is partly because of the cost of services, for which she would have to pay, but Frau Jakob also cannot think of any useful services that she might need. As with many of the other carers, being in sole charge has made it difficult for her to step outside the situation and assess her own needs, which she is not very skilled in detecting. Her own definition of the situation closes off help, isolates her, and delays contact with services in the first place. As she does not allow any professional into her confidence, she also shuts herself off from other forms of assistance, for example in her neighbourhood. With the new care insurance and the potentially expanding role of domiciliary and other support services, a more proactive approach among service providers to support informal carers might benefit carers like Frau Jakob. Persistent and sensitive attempts at intervention might have led her to be able to accept more assistance, although a substantial change seems unlikely, given her emotional investment in her caring activity. In the cases of Frau Hamann, Frau Hegemann and Frau Luchtig, more offers of services could make a difference, in that they might break up their isolation. In the case of Frau Luchtig, a wider range of services might allow her to persuade her mother to take advantage of them.

Most of the carers we interviewed were ambivalent about carer groups, finding such 'public' association uncomfortable and difficult. This may be understandable, given an essentially private definition of caring tasks. Frau Alexander, who is so successful in negotiating with authorities and has many years of experience, refuses to participate in a carer group, which she regards as being of little help on a practical level. Emotionally, she cannot articulate her own traumas, and listening to those of others may be unbearable. She has always operated on her own, and because of the lack of social support during the initial phase of caring, lacks the skills and experience to share her anxieties with other parents. Her absence deprives other parents of a source of great experience and skill, and she herself loses the opportunity to explore other dimensions of caring through the support of the group. It is clear that public meetings do not seem to be the right step for those who are only used to operating in the private sphere.

Lack of outside contact delays planning for caring beyond home-based care. Among carers of older children, there is little thinking about future living arrangements. Care of elders is regarded as a family affair until the end; this is reinforced by the high cost of residential and nursing accommodation. Reactive services and advice, which do not have access to the private sphere unless invited, cannot easily help carers along the path of decision making. This creates crisis situations, where decisions have to be taken on the spur of the moment. Frau Jakob's sudden decision to take her husband home from hospital occurred without consultation, with disastrous consequences for her quality of life for the next two and a half years.

Conclusion

The German situation is characterised by the pervasive influence of the values of traditional family politics in West German welfare society. In many ways, caring for disabled and frail dependants magnifies the consequences of gendered divisions between the public and private spheres. Those carers who allow themselves to be absorbed by these structures can become enclosed within the private sphere, dependent on close family relations and family support. This dependency can produce crises which trap the female carer in very difficult circumstances. At the same time, caring carries a powerful identity and status of its own, making it a valid choice for West German women. For those carers who are able to remain connected to the outside world, caring in the informal sphere offers scope for innovation and development, and provides a powerful basis for identity formation and bold life choices.

Considered within the wider context of social change, the informal sphere of caring offers an interesting commentary on the process of modernisation. Vester (1993) argues that West German post-industrial society has been subject to a number of setbacks in recent years, which have reversed processes of social integration and created "lines of social conflict" (pp 4-5). He argues that this process acts as a counterpoint to the liberating and progressive opportunities which arise from the process of modernisation. While modernisation contributes to dissolving old social orders and furthers structural changes towards the individualisation of lifestyles and the pluralisation of social milieus, the new lines of conflict create 'losers' and 'winners'. For the purposes of our study, it is interesting that Vester identifies the seat of reform and innovation in milieus at the margins of the social structure, for example in the self-help movement and the alternative milieus, particularly among lower and middle-class milieus. However, their impact for social innovation and modernisation remains limited, blocked by the influence of the greater group of political and economic élites.

This analysis helps to explain why it is so difficult for the informal sphere of caring to allow greater openness to the wider social engagement of carers. Alternatives to the traditional family in the private sphere are not filtering through to carers in a consistent way. Independent living movements are developing alternative living arrangements; however, their influence is limited to a comparatively small field, and the political influence of the disability movement has not penetrated mainstream political discourse as it has in Britain, for instance. Caring remains part of the private family institutional structure, and there is little indication that it will become politicised in the same way as it is in Britain. There are few political incentives to change this fundamental pattern of caring, as the most pressing political problem – the financing of expensive residential and nursing care provision – has been resolved from within through the introduction of care insurance. The most innovative interventions come from within the private caring realm, from individuals who for reasons of biography or circumstance fall outside the normative framework of care. Innovative developments also occur within the large welfare organisations, which experiment with alternative measures.

The successful strategies of carers such as Frau Luchtig, Frau Mahler and Frau Alexander, of opening their private spheres up to the public and social worlds for additional support, circumvent the endemic problems of isolation and loneliness. The problem with these carer strategies is that they remain individual solutions, based on essentially personal resources. The developments and changes these women experience remain private victories, unique to their own circumstances. Their significance as examples of an excitingly different approach to informal care is lost to other carers.

Notes

[1] Ostner (1993, p 100 ff) cites parental leave and the Erziehungsgeld policies as two major reasons for the comparatively slow change to the continued (economic)

dependency of mothers in the West German family unit. Erziehungsgeld (an extended, monthly flat-rate childcare allowance, payable in addition to child benefit) was meant to soften the impact of loss of earnings for either parent who stayed at home. Available up to two years after the birth of the child, it became a powerful incentive for married women to stay at home. In 1986, 94% of working mothers took both parental leave and this flat-rate benefit.

[2] In European comparisons, German men are more conservative in their attitudes to the division of labour among couples: 59% prefer their partners to be homemakers, against 31% who would like their partners to be working. The European average is 43% for homemakers and 47% for working women. Overall, West Germans prefer partial equality or traditional roles in the division of labour (66%) to equality (26%). The European average is 54% and 41% respectively (source: Becker, 1989).

[3] The married earnings allowance in Germany is much higher than in Britain. Ironically, childless couples benefit most from the married person's allowance, because they can split the allowance to maximise tax breaks on individual incomes. In Germany, this widens the gap between single mothers and childless, married women (Clasen and Freeman, 1994).

[4] The project started at a time of intense public debate about creating a separate care insurance to address the increasingly high private and public costs of the care requirements of older people.

[5] Four years after the introduction of care insurance, German commentators are already talking about a financial crisis in the scheme: the German health ministry is expecting a financial shortfall of DM 750,000,000 – more if benefits are raised (quoted in BerlinOnLine, 12 August 2000).

THREE

East Germany – the push out of the home

Introduction

The East German system of state socialism provided a markedly different framework for caring as compared with West Germany. After 40 years of separate existence, the two German regimes diverged not only in their administrative arrangements and underlying social principles, but also in their social infrastructures of family, neighbourhood and workplace. Unification, which started in 1990, imposed the family-centred and pluralised system of the social state on a quite different terrain.

Of the five caring situations presented in this chapter, three date from many years before unification, and two began in the turmoil of that period. Since the new system of welfare was still a fledgling in 1992 when the interviews were conducted, all five sets of caring arrangements and strategies were strongly framed by GDR society. The case studies and the interviews with welfare personnel both convey the experience for East Germans of living in the GDR, and the hopes and fears brought by unification.

Writing and thinking about the GDR involves negotiating between Eastern and Western perspectives, and what often seems the absence of an authentic view. Merkel (1994) maintains that women's experiences have been no better captured in Western-dominated discourse after unification than they were under the old regime. This enhances the importance of these case studies, which provide eloquent testimony to the experience of being a carer in East Germany before and during unification, and the personal and public struggles involved. The cases are based on full and heartfelt accounts. The carers responded boldly to the opportunity to talk, both for themselves and as representatives of the hidden constituency of carers. It often seemed that this was the first time they had been addressed as carers, 'caring' being completely unacknowledged in East German society[1]. There was also a sense in which they were using the interview to bear testimony for East German experience as a whole, with love and loathing, and were glad to be offered a space in which to speak outside the hegemony of West German discourse[2].

Unification

Several West German commentators came to regret the speed of unification: the Berlin Wall fell in November 1989, East German elections were held in March 1990, the currency unified in June, the Unification Treaty signed in November, and all-German elections held in December 1990. Criticisms of the West German system, which had been widely voiced during the 1980s, were suddenly dropped, so that an opportunity for reform of the Federal system was missed. Nor was there any time for Western social policy experts, few of whom had even set foot in East Germany, to familiarise themselves with its intricate systems of informal support. The opportunity to graft on rather than to override and replace was therefore lost (Backhaus-Maul and Olk, 1993; Lorenz, 1994). Yet interviews with East German welfare experts in 1991 and 1992 showed their determination to hold onto some of the valued features of East German 'ways of doing things', and to the innovative reform ideas (such as shared parenting) which flourished in the period immediately following the fall of the Berlin Wall. These aspirations were as strong among lower level personnel as among the more senior. Follow-up discussions in 1993 showed the frailty of such hopes in the face of the 'steamroller' of West German administrative and financial imperatives. The one-stop 'polyclinics' which existed in many workplaces and localities were a case in point. They provided immediate access to on-the-spot specialist health services, from a staff of 20 to 30 doctors (Hildebrandt, 1994, p 23; Bradley Scharf, 1984). But they simply did not fit and could not be financed by the West German health insurance system, which is based on privately owned practices.

Social policy in East Germany

We begin with the centralised character of the GDR welfare system, its rootedness in the workplace, its relative marginalisation of local government and neighbourhood organisation, and some features of its policies towards elderly and disabled people and towards women. We also describe the newly established welfare organisations and the health service-based social stations through which we gained access to the carers in 1992.

Workplace-based services

The centralisation and tight integration of economic and social policy in the GDR aimed to serve industry and win legitimacy at home and abroad (Adams, 1990). Unification posed an immense problem of personnel, since the 'cadre' administration which had been used to implementing orders from above was now required to operate a federalist system of professional accountability (Lorenz, 1994, p 166). Closures and marketisation swept away entire swathes of health, housing and social facilities in the workplace enterprises. And whereas in the GDR full employment and subsidies for food, rent and transport had virtually erased the phenomenon of 'social security cases', (Backhaus-Maul and Olk, 1993, p 307), after unification the marketising of production and consumption caused social assistance claims to soar. In 1993, 'real' unemployment, undisguised by early retirement, short-time working and job training, was calculated to be 37% (Lorenz, 1994, p 166). The state-run health services had to be reconfigured to fit the West German system, in which health insurance funds reign supreme.

At local government level, the contrasts were equally great. For while West German federalism places service provision in regional and local government, in East Germany the key locus lay in local factories and workplaces, where the Socialist Unity Party (SED) was the main organiser. This marginalised local government, but also weakened party scrutiny over it. Local councils, supported by the mass organisations for children, youth, women and elderly people, had the task of compensating for the underfunding of communal services by mobilising voluntary effort through neighbourhood committees and tenants' associations. Such citizen participation, widely seen as 'citizen exploitation', was used to renovate old people's flats; build and maintain playgrounds, public gardens and open spaces; and collect metal, glass and paper for recycling. The key providers of meals-on-wheels, home visits and home-help services for disabled and housebound people were younger retired people, organised through *Volkssolidarität* (People's Solidarity). Such services received token remuneration, and home helps a low rate of pay (Chamberlayne, 1990a; 1995). One of the factors which enabled the churches to survive was their role in organising services for those outside the orbit of the enterprises, such as more severely disabled or very elderly people.

Social policy expansion in the 1970s and 1980s brought major benefits, especially in maternity leave and childcare provision[3]. Whereas health and education had been prioritised in the 1950s and 1960s, attention shifted in the 1980s to the appalling state of housing (Michalsky, 1984, pp 254-8; Krisch, 1985). In some areas, local meetings were held to discuss new housing projects and renovation schemes, but these only exposed the use of house building and housing allocation for purposes of labour recruitment and reward, and the consequent neglect of all other groups[4]. The lack of central heating, inside toilets, baths and hot water remained highest among older age groups (in 1989, 18% of dwellings generally had no bath or shower, 24% no inside toilet, and 53% no central heating (Backhaus-Maul and Olk, 1993, p 317)). This meant that domiciliary service might well involve slopping out (in old blocks of flats toilets were often on half-landings) and carrying coal for fires (possibly up many flights of stairs). Winters are very cold in East Germany, as is general in Central Europe.

The inadequacy of local government resourcing led to innovative partnership 'contracts' between enterprises and local councils, the extended use of enterprise facilities for meals-on-wheels and transport, and improved coordination among services. An internationally eminent gerontologist in Leipzig referred with pride to the system of 'komplexe Betreuung' (complex care) for elderly people, which coordinated the services of 11 diverse agencies, under the direction of the Ministry of Health, with parallel groups at regional and neighbourhood level (Hildebrandt, 1994, p 19). He admitted that there was a problem of who would take real responsibility, but said that the key frustration was the lack of resources.

Women and family policy

The family was central to postwar reconstruction in both parts of Germany. But whereas West Germany's social policy cast women's roles firmly in the domestic sphere, East Germany's policy of the 'family for socialism' claimed women's emancipation through labour, with state provision to relieve domestic burdens (Chamberlayne, 1994). These different perspectives resulted in dramatic differences in provision and life patterns. For example, while about 70% of childrearing costs in East Germany were covered by family subsidies, only 25% of such costs were publicly borne in West Germany. And while only 3% of East German women espoused a full-time housewife role, the comparable figure in West Germany was 25% (Gerhard, 1991-92, p 23; Althammer and Pfaff, 1999).

Distinguishing periods of social policy helps in delineating a generational profile of women's experience, which has relevance for caring. According to Penrose (1990), the period 1946-65 focused on integrating women into the labour force and in protecting mothers. Key concerns in 1963-72, following the mass exodus of qualified people and the building of the Berlin Wall, lay in higher education and professional qualifications for women. The third period, 1971-89, introduced 'Muttipolitik' (mummy politics), which sought to aid the balancing of career and family. In all three periods most women worked full-time, so that by the late 1980s three generations had grown up with working mothers.

Each generation of mothers combined work and family responsibilities in different ways. The first generation had to make individual and private arrangements for childcare, and half of those who resumed full-time work (93%) took up to eight years out of the labour market when their children were young (Trappe, 1995, p 119). Mothers born around 1940 worked more continuously, although most of their children were still cared for privately in their early years in the late 1960s (Trappe, 1995, p 122). This generation greatly appreciated the extension of childcare provision. For the third generation, born in the 1950s, matters became more contradictory. The GDR was by now the only socialist state to provide both full pre-school provision and generous 'baby year' allowances (Bertram, 1992, p 28; Hildebrandt, 1994, p 20). This gave women a real choice of whether to work or not, but implicitly recognised the importance of early mothering. Those who stayed at home became conflicted about their roles, felt isolated, and experienced public resentment against their 'privileges' and a backlash restrengthening of the traditional division of labour (Ferree, 1993, p 109; Dölling, 1994).

Women's groups which sprang up in 1989-90 focused on the disenfranchising nature of the 'father' and 'guardian' state. Demanding more self-determination and voice for women, they expressed no desire to separate from men, appealing rather for men's rights and responsibilities in parenting, especially in step- and lone-parenting, and for improved cooperation between men and women. In West Germany, by contrast, autonomy both from men and from the state, and self-determination in marriage relations, have been prime issues in women's politics. These differences have made cooperation among women from East and West Germany difficult since unification (Young, 1994).

Self-help groups

Unification led to a rich discussion concerning informal cultures and networks. The West German writer, Claus Offe (1991), feared that welfare reform would run aground in East Germany for lack of social infrastructures, while East German writers linked the mushrooming of independent organisations in 1989-90 with the prior culture of trust in work and house collectives and garden associations (Wielgohs, 1993). For Pollack (1992), the meaningless discourse and rituals in the public sphere meant that the private sphere gained ground as a site for innovation, engagement and empathy, for achieving a sense of self, and fulfilling a need for communication. The culture of 'helping one another' formed around informal exchanges of goods and services, in lieu of public or market provision; informal networking circumvented officialdom, and gained access to a preferred school or special medical treatment. Pollack points to the narrow provincialism of informal networks, and their instrumental rather than genuinely collectivist nature.

As long as retired workers in the GDR were mobile, they benefited from workplace facilities such as health clinics and canteens, and social, sports and holiday activities. Many attendant and reception positions (in offices, museums and toilets) were kept for retired people. Workplaces were obliged to protect 20% of their employment positions for disabled people, and disabled children and young people classified as 'educable' (förderfähig) received special educational and vocational training. Transport was not provided, however, and provision was particularly inadequate for adults with more severe learning difficulties. One informant calculated that one-third of mothers of such young adults over 30 were at home as carers, and that workplace closures meant that 1,300 daytime places were now needed in Leipzig, while only 360 existed.

Association with a workplace involved not just an independent income, but sociability and a sense of belonging, from past or present membership of a 'work collective'. Intended as a means of political indoctrination and control, work 'brigades' of 10-12 colleagues became a key locus of social solidarity and friendship. Böckmann-Schewe et al (1995, p 219) refer to the 'conspiratorial irony' with which women workers responded to directives from above, and the implanting of the work collective in the safety of community and a culture of solidarity. Members of work collectives knew about each others' family affairs, often went on holidays and social outings together, and shared babysitting and weekend meals. In a private interview, Detlev Pollack (an East German theologian and sociologist) argued that over-politicisation of public discourse meant that personal communication and intimacy had to spill out somewhere, and that the workplace generated among workers a sense of collective strength of being needed.

Party leader claims to socialist superiority in satisfying human needs enraged those most dependent on welfare services, and groups of elderly and disabled people were prominent in the demonstrations and grassroots activities which marked events in the Spring of 1989-90. These groups, which previously had not been formally organised, lacked the international profile of the dissident groups on peace, human rights and the environment. Their shared understandings of the failures and hypocrisies of the system, and their informal networks of mutual support and information, nevertheless amounted to a 'quiet social movement' which then burst into life (Hofmann, 1991). In 1992, the Disability Association (Behindertenverband) in Leipzig, an umbrella group for a range of independent initiatives, employed 33 people, half of whom were disabled. The Disability Office from Leipzig's city council ran a work group of 33 independent and self-help organisations, the Office of Health supported 26 self-help groups for elderly people, and the city ran a 60-strong Committee for Elderly People. These groups were mobilised by opposition to both GDR conditions and the losses of unification.

The organisation of domiciliary services

At the time of our interviews, the reorganising of the welfare system was still underway. The city council was eager to off-load nurseries, residential homes and day centres, while the welfare organisations, still finding their feet, were resisting taking on too many new responsibilities too quickly.

The social stations which organised domiciliary services for housebound people had been functioning since September 1990. Community nurses, previously from the health service or the churches, had been allocated to 55 districts in the city, each with a population of 20,000-40,000, under one of the five new welfare organisations (for details of the welfare organisations see p 29; there was no Jewish welfare organisation in Leipzig). Home-help and meals-on-wheels services were being distributed likewise, although some of these services were still provided by Volkssolidarität. Equipment from the rehabilitation and various mobile services had been privatised. The staffing of social stations was variable. An experienced community nurse might lead three to 10 trained nurses, three to five care assistants, between two and 25 home helps, one to four clerical staff, two drivers possibly, and up to 10 Zivis. Noticeably lacking were social workers, Sozialpädagogen, counsellors and psychologists – professions which barely existed in the GDR – although many felt that the three-year nurse training included 'everything'. The lack of training among the previously quasi-voluntary home helps was much criticised, but so was the 'cowboy' character of the new six- to 20-week courses for care assistants in the care of elderly people (*Altenpfleger*).

In 1992, clear differences in attitudes and capacities of the five welfare organisations were apparent. Leaders of the Protestant and Catholic churches, the Innere Mission and Caritas, felt embarrassed by the new mantle of welfare, firstly because of the fundamentally secular nature of East German society. (Church officials estimated membership figures at 20% Protestant and 4% Catholic in East Germany; this compares with 47% and 44% respectively in West Germany (Madeley, 1991, p 35). Secondly they considered their role as primarily spiritual, and thirdly they valued their own forms of training and their more personalised approach.) Under unification they were obliged to take over whole institutions and bodies of staff, adopt standard norms in the costing of nursing, treatment and basic care tasks, and comply with bureaucratic procedures for gaining nursing-home places for clients, certification of particular levels of disability and different health insurance payments. All this jeopardised the humanist and spiritual aspects of their work, which necessitated continuity of staffing and much time for talk and 'sitting together'.

Volkssolidarität, which had been the main provider of home helps, meals-on-wheels (actually meals-in-the-basket, since they were carried on foot) and good neighbour work, stood tarred by association with the old regime, even of being 'terrorist', since it had sent funds to Nicaragua. Opinions voiced in interviews varied wildly: it did an excellent job, based on committed work and sensitive networks; it was full of corruption and petty theft; it consisted of unprofessional busybodies and relied on embarrassing door-to-door collections (Chamberlayne, 1995). Eventually, in 1993, Volkssolidarität gained the right to take on contracts for welfare work. But it was hampered by a number of problems such as its large body of untrained staff to whom it owed loyalty, its restriction to services to elderly people, and its lack of a culture of open accountability.

The main constituency of the DPWV umbrella association (see p 29) lay in the myriad independent and innovative initiatives which had sprung up in 1989-90. Many of these organisations opposed Volkssolidarität joining the DPWV in 1993. Its dominant size and the greater experience of its functionaries placed it well to take on regional and city-level posts for the DPWV, whereas the newer initiatives were struggling with bureaucratised procedures, funding, reliance on short-term job-creation posts, and the syphoning off of their main activists, untainted by association with the previous regime, to more secure jobs in local government.

The Red Cross existed as a membership organisation in the GDR. Mainly based in workplaces, but also in neighbourhoods, it had specialised in first aid, health and safety, and ambulance services, and lacked professional experience in running health or social services. Like Volkssolidarität, it suffered from association with the old regime, and its membership had diminished from 20,000 to 1,000. In East Germany, the Workers' Welfare Organisation (AWO), firmly rooted in worker milieus in West Germany, had no roots at all. The Sozialdemokratische Partei Deutschlands (SPD) had been banned in East Germany since the early 1930s, and the longstanding hostility between communist and social democratic loyalties still seemed to hang in the air in the 1990s. Both AWO and the Red Cross adopted an administrative approach (Angerhausen et al, 1993, p 22), with little reflection at senior level about how the new welfare systems might address the particular needs of East German society. Staff in the social stations, by contrast, talked at length about how housing conditions, family and work patterns, and the new fear of going out affected the management of domiciliary services in East Germany[5]. Like the church and Volkssolidarität officials, they valued the humanism and culture of mutual help which had characterised social life in East Germany, and were determined to uphold good practice. As one staff member put it: "We still do a lot of things, I must say, just as we used to before". Speaking of the need to allow time to talk, a Red Cross nurse said, "They [patients] just want to get it off their chest sometimes (von der Seele reden)".

Unification brought many improvements: equipment for residential care and incontinence, disability workshops, better mobility and transport, and a diversity of specialist training for staff working with children with learning difficulties. On the other hand, many facilities and aids were expensive, with bureaucratic procedures for establishing access and eligibility. For all their determination to maintain 'the good things' from the old system, social stations and welfare organisations were too preoccupied with survival and management to dedicate time to lobbying for reform. The 'old' organisations like Volkssolidarität and the Red Cross were more concerned with gaining political acceptance than challenging the incoming system. Nevertheless, there was quite a ferment of innovation and reflective thinking, also from the dense pattern of twinning arrangements between West and East German towns and agencies.

The East German cases

The carers were used to going out to work full-time and taking children out daily to crèches and schools. They habitually used informal contacts and networks to negotiate around the system and solve the problems of everyday life. While the West German partners tended to play a complementary role based on a traditional division of labour, the East German partners often shared intimate and routine caring tasks. Involvement in the outside world might require sharing at home, and the personal courage entailed in social interactions with strangers and confronting officialdom also necessitated a strong home base. The outer-connectedness of most East German carers brought them in contact with different perspectives, so that – despite an absence of official discourse concerning disability – the carers were challenged in their views, leading to greater reflexivity on difference and disabled people's rights.

We only present five cases in this chapter, because we only came across one case of 'retreat into the private sphere'. That carer is an older man, who in building a fortress around the care of his wife, seems at least partially motivated by resistance to the collectivised system. We begin with examples of a more characteristic outward dynamic among East German carers, which we call 'trawling the social sphere'. This impulse is also strongly present in the third category of 'transition' cases, which are torn between traditional home-based and outward-oriented roles. Both the carers in this category encountered the challenge of caring in the period of unification.

Trawling the social sphere

The first two cases have long experiences of bringing up disabled children. Both have been involved on an ongoing basis in seeking out services of their choice in defiance of official directions. Using informal networks, they gain advice from sympathetic professionals and from others in a similar situation. Their contacts extend to the West, from where they acquire specialist equipment and information about treatments which they can conduct at home. Their complex and innovative arrangements are constantly changing and being renegotiated. Even when they stop work for purposes of caring, they remain active outside the home. Their caring experiences lead to a striking degree of personal development.

Frau Meissner's strength derives from her skills in mobilising support – from her family, from professionals, and from her ex-husband, even though he is now remarried and has another child. Despite sacrificing her personal life for her daughter, Frau Meissner has gained a great sense of personal fulfilment and adventure through caring. The Grüns are a young couple who have been caring for seven years. Professionally qualified and belonging to a church milieu, they interweave a complex web of care from both public and private spheres. Their main resource lies in their close relationship as a couple, which they use both in dealing with the public world and in understanding their young son. In both cases, the carers show marked respect for the individuality of the disabled young person. Frau Meissner has acquired this attitude through the challenge of her daughter's adolescence, but also by participating in integrated education and encountering the principle of independent living, while the Grüns are influenced by the deep humanism and person-centredness of their religion.

Frau Meissner

Frau Meissner has a daughter of 20 who has been partially paralysed from birth and uses a wheelchair. Initially a single parent, she has always been Katrin's principal carer. She has also been strongly supported by her family, and then by her husband, who is Katrin's father. The father has a new family, but continues to give assistance.

Frau Meissner gives up her job in industrial administration to look after Katrin who, because of her incontinence, would otherwise be placed in residential care. By active negotiation, Frau Meissner finds a succession of schools which will accept Katrin and allow Frau Meissner to stay nearby to help her.

Following the offer of vocational training for Katrin in Berlin, the parents succeed in gaining an apprenticeship in a local public service. They provide the daily transport themselves. Zivis give Katrin lifts for leisure purposes. Frau Meissner is active in helping with school outings, and with discos and sports for disabled youngsters. Recently she has taken Katrin and two disabled friends to the United States (US) on holiday, and hopes to repeat the experience. When a properly adapted flat for Katrin and her boyfriend comes through, Frau Meissner will try to live nearby.

Frau Meissner's own biography is told through an account of her daughter's disability. Her adult life is exclusively devoted to her daughter's needs, but in that process she has developed remarkable capacities. Rather than remaining locked into the cost and pain of her caring commitment, she appreciates her life as successful in other areas.

Frau Meissner has a relationship with Katrin's father for two years before she becomes pregnant. She lives with her parents and her boyfriend is a student in another town, with his military service still before him. By the time they marry a couple of years later, Frau Meissner has established a role as sole carer, backed in all the practical tasks of caring and carrying by her older siblings, who are childless, and by her mother. She arranges for Katrin to receive mainstream education, accompanying her to school in order to deal with her incontinence, and she goes on school trips, lifting Katrin up all the stairs, "leaving all the men behind", as she puts it. Some years later, Frau Meissner is offered a permanent job as a school nurse, a position she greatly enjoys. In the process of defying the authorities, she has developed considerable organising and campaigning talents.

Part of Frau Meissner's strength lies in her capacity to ask for help. Faced with pressure to put Katrin in a residential home, and even offered a job there herself, she gains the backing of headteachers and other local influentials who themselves have disabled children. She persuades teachers to meet the tram every morning to lift down the wheelchair, and makes herself useful in the school. By 1989, she has imported several wheelchairs from West Germany, one brightly coloured, one arriving in parts through the post. She appreciates the help she receives, and is full of praise for the ready offers of help throughout her visit to the US with Katrin and two other disabled friends, one also using a wheelchair.

When we considered the beginning of her biography, we anticipated that Frau Meissner's emotional dependence on Katrin would greatly inhibit the development and autonomy of both of them. But it has worked out otherwise. Frau Meissner's story is one of overcoming self-subordination through a fight for someone else. Nevertheless, Frau Meissner's interview suggests complex issues of interdependency between mother and daughter, and of unresolved issues around partnerships.

Frau Meissner has lived through her daughter, at the expense of her marriage and further relationships, yet she has enabled her daughter to gain a degree of autonomy and has opened up otherwise unlikely possibilities for her own life. She has used interdependence to gain her own social independence; she has gained an interdependent kind of autonomy. Katrin's father was excluded from her early life by the delay in the marriage and by the close family constellation on Frau Meissner's side. It may be that Frau Meissner's resistance to residential care was motivated by her own personal dependency needs, but also that Katrin's attendance at a normal school has facilitated her autonomy. Zivis have become friends of both of them and provide Katrin with transport. Katrin visits clubs, has trained in the post office, is learning to drive and wants to share a flat with her boyfriend. Frau Meissner expects to go on living near to Katrin. Perhaps she already has a model of this in her contact with her husband's new family – they share the same garden, much to the neighbours' puzzlement.

Frau Meissner's self-effacement shows through in the structure of the interview. She repeatedly shies away from any discussion of herself or her divorce, but in both interviews, in the last few pages, she suddenly and articulately pours out her own feelings:

> Of course I must say, for me personally, for me alone, a lot has been forsaken. The divorce with her father was connected with it. Not that he doesn't like her, that I always put her first [pause], but then I couldn't change my spots.

She continues that the divorce was not stormy, it took two minutes. She was upset, but had her job and the flat, and decided to begin again. "But in the final analysis I made the same mistake again, I only considered Katrin". She explains that now she feels she has established such 'perfection' in her life, she doesn't need anyone else. She indicates that she has had plenty of offers of partnerships.

Her answers to questions about the option of putting Katrin in a home remain uneasy, however. The nervousness of the interviewer suggests that she is picking up on Frau Meissner's guardedness: "And there was never a question that Katrin, well you never would have sent Katrin boarding, well it was clear to you from the beginning, that Katrin lives with you?". There is a pause before Frau Meissner replies, "Well it just happened like that", whereupon the interviewer takes fright: "Or was it through external circumstances?". At the end of the second interview, Frau Meissner indicates that the decision did and still does trouble her, though the particular context lies in worries about her pension as a single woman:

> if I had perhaps given her up to Wermsdorf (the residential home), then everything would have been different, but I didn't want to and couldn't manage it and so it is, nothing can be changed about that.

The Grüns

> Frau Grün is 18 and training as a nurse when Jo is born in 1985; Herr Grün
> is 24 and studying theology. Jo is born with a spinal deformity which was not
> picked up by ultrasound, and has a drain for hydrocephalus. His parents
> tackle his physical disabilities through an extensive regime of exercises, which
> they learn via contacts in West Germany.
>
> Despite using a special wheelchair, Jo goes to a conventional kindergarten
> for three or four hours a day, thanks to a private arrangement. He will soon
> move on to a school. Only his parents and one friend can empty Jo's bladder
> correctly, by pressure on the abdomen, so one of them has to be present
> every three or four hours. The parents' working hours are fitted around
> each other, and they can rarely go out as a couple. Frau Grün relies on
> public transport because she cannot drive.

The opening exchanges of the interview richly anticipate the key themes
which are to follow. The interviewer feels awkward, because the couple
present themselves together and resist the open format. At one level,
their conducting of the interview together and involving their child is a
sign of their democratic partnership and family values. On closer
interpretation, their insistence on being questioned rather than speaking
freely, their determination to focus on Jo's development rather than on
their experiences as carers, and their repeated turn-taking and talk with
Jo during the interview are all means of avoiding straying into more
personalised narrative. An interview is itself situated at the interface of
public and private worlds, and the Grüns' approach corresponds with
their way of dealing with the public world and protecting their privacy.
Controlling while working across the public–private divide characterises
their approach to caring. It is a defensive cultural form which seems
rather particular to East German society, or perhaps to the dissident church
milieu to which they belong. Their case contrasts with the Mahlers in
West Germany, who also use their professionalism to transcend the public–
private divide, but without having to defend their privacy.

The Grüns' negotiations are skilful and diplomatic, while the interviewer
is thoroughly unnerved:

Interviewer: So could you tell me, how it began, I, I don't know
                 very much.

Frau Grün:	I thought this was based on firm questions...
Interviewer:	No, not at all.
Frau Grün:	... on some concrete questions.
Interviewer:	I only have, if I get stuck or something, I note it down, make some points. So you can talk now about whatever you want, so there's, there are no points, no points.

The interviewer complies, directing the couple to a chronological and medical account of Jo's illness and development. Each partner picks up on difficult passages from the other, whether to prevent the other from straying too far into the personal arena or to make a complementary point, and the interviewer mostly shies away from addressing emotionally difficult territory in subsequent questions, even when, in spite of themselves, the Grüns create clear openings for this.

The couple use their professional backgrounds and informal contacts to reject and fight against some services, while gaining access to and carefully monitoring and maintaining control over others. Their account is structured around the typical GDR duality of 'desertion/lack of interest by the system' and 'helpful informal contacts and individuals'. In the early stages they receive little or no help from medical professionals and have to push hard for progress for Jo. Frau Grün recalls the feeling of being deserted following the birth:

> Well after four weeks, it wasn't quite healed yet, but because I was a nurse, still training at that time, we could take him home, they just showed us a bit more. And because he is paraplegic, he needs to have his bladder emptied through pressure, well, they demonstrated it briefly and then we stood there alone in empty fields, there wasn't much.

Herr Grün speaks of the callous doctor who advises them to accept their bad luck and have another child, and the 'friendly but helpless' surgeon who doesn't know how to relate to parents who ask questions. He says that the expectation of passivity belonged to the political culture of the regime.

For a long period, the Grüns are passed from clinic to clinic in four medical appointments a week. Progress only comes through personal contacts and appeals, and by speeding up a referral to the social-paediatric centre, where the specialist staff include psychologists; here they find real help and commitment. Jo is by now four months old:

> She gave us advice, she knew how to do something practical. He wasn't allowed to lie on his side and the water content of his head was controlled through tilting. And if it is tilted too much, then the plates collapse and if it's too flat, then the brain pressure increases. And, if you're not too careful with little infants, with very little infants, everything grows incorrectly, because everything is mixed up. And the operation scar was here, and we put something underneath and other such very little things, and he couldn't swallow.

The same paediatrician regularly monitors Jo, to determine whether he is capable of attending school. If not, he would be designated 'ineducable' and sent to a residential home. To avoid this, the parents implement a method of physiotherapy which involves monthly training for themselves and half-an-hour's training three times a day for Jo. It is painful and he cries a lot. They force him to eat and drink to avoid a return to hospital. Later on they switch to another intensive method, and now use a more relaxed, 'mixed' approach.

First through necessity and later by their successful experiences in negotiating around different institutions, they become experts in the management of Jo's disability. They delay his designation to a special crèche for severely disabled children, and then restrict his attendance to half days. They win the personal interest and responsiveness of particular professionals in Jo and his situation, and gain access to an integrated kindergarten. He is the first paraplegic child to be thus accepted:

Frau Grün: Well I had heard about conventional kindergartens, that they had sometimes children – I had heard about a child with learning disability, but I couldn't imagine it with Jo in the wheelchair. I went there and asked and it was already in the autumn [of 1989, the year of the Wende], things were changing, and they had thought about it and I came along at the right moment. They said yes, wanted to see Jo first, and they have a young nursery nurse [laughs] and she is very good with him.

While they are highly appreciative of Jo's social talents and 'winning character', of his fantasy life and ability to tell himself long stories, his musicality, and his responsiveness to their friends and activities, they are struggling with their own criteria of 'normality'. They realise that more contact with parents of disabled children might be helpful, as the interviewer tentatively suggests, and that they will have to break out of their existing private sphere and points of reference. Herr Grün is reluctant to join organisations following his membership of the Young Pioneers (the Communist children's organisation) and the organised youth movement, and Frau Grün has been preoccupied with her course.

They feel that their perception of child development is distorted by their experience of Jo, and are pained to see that other children learn in a few moments what they can spend six months or two years teaching Jo:

Herr Grün: You can see it when you have any four year old telling
              you something in the kindergarten, they have done
              this and that and then there was this, and they nearly
              fall over each other with talking and he can't do it,
              can't do it, can't reproduce these simple activities
              coherently. He has the pictures in his head and can't
              put them together. These are things which one can
              only comprehend after a while.

Frau Grün: The success stories are simply very rare. Otherwise
              one is perhaps a bit proud of one's child and so it's
              hard. Because, that's something missing, because one
              makes all the more effort and all the less comes out.

There are hints of problems in the closeness of their relationship. They have maintained a wide circle of friends and visitors, and continue to go on walking, biking and taking seaside holidays, destroying three prams in the process, but at the same time depend utterly on each other. Frau Grün admits the "horror" she initially felt at the whole day being taken up in caring, and finds the situation only manageable "together or not at all". She is stressed if her husband is away. Jo's disability has 'welded' them together, but perhaps excessively so. They feel that by having a disabled member the whole family is 'disabled'.

Their own families are barely mentioned. Frau Grün associates with her brother, but her mother is on a *Mitleidschiene* (sympathy track) which jars with their strategy, which is to 'normalise' both Jo's abilities and their situation. They are supported by friends rather than family, and talk with guarded enthusiasm about the future. They intend to have other children and are open to the idea of a boarding school in about five years' time, provided that Jo can manage with a catheter. They envisage models of group living and communities for disabled people, so that Jo could become independent from them, though the unclear nature of his developmental problems makes them hesitant about what would be possible. The Wende has brought him a wonderful new wheelchair, large and generous financial benefits, and more varied and intensive therapies and possibilities, "if they don't do away with everything – they're cutting things like crazy". The improvements, greater for children than for adults, are not for everyone anyway. More immediately, Herr Grün, now qualified as a pastor, will only accept a parish with access to good schooling for Jo. Meanwhile, Frau Grün is considering a degree in social pedagogy, which has a strong element of psychology.

'Home is best' – retreat into the private sphere

Among our East German carers, only one remains locked in the private sphere, resisting the offer of outside services. Herr Speyer's proud self-sufficiency defies the tenets and practices of East German welfare, at both formal and informal levels. The patriarchal element in his strategy of assuming full control and management of his wife's illness is perhaps reinforced by his experience of running a private taxi business in the special culture of the private sector. Though beleaguered in an almost fully collectivised economy, the private sector of handicrafts and retail services was resilient in East Germany. It flourished following greater political recognition in the 1980s.

Herr Speyer

Herr Speyer's wife is disabled through epilepsy. The epilepsy begins following the birth of her older daughter 38 years ago and is exacerbated by the birth of a second daughter 10 years later. From then onwards, Herr Speyer increasingly takes on caring as well as household tasks, refusing the option of residential care. Nowadays, he is rarely able to work in his taxi business because his wife needs constant supervision. Two recent strokes have virtually removed her awareness of her surroundings and any sense of safety. Her every move has to be watched, and if Herr Speyer needs to go out he ties her in her bed.

Herr Speyer's narrative is confined to his caring experience. His marriage, the birth of his daughter and his wife's epilepsy all occurred in the same year, and it seems as if his life before and outside of the caring commitment has fallen away. He presents himself as a lifelong carer, who loyally and single-handedly copes with an ever-more confining situation:

> ... and I was told then, 15 years ago, when it got worse, what I would have to face [one-second pause] because with each fit, brain cells die. Well, it got worse with each year [two-second pause]. I have been cooking for about ten years [two-second pause].... I think, I knew it from the beginning [two-second pause] another man would have disappeared after two, three years [two-second pause]. I said, I won't do that, I won't spoil the whole of my life. We were married at the age of 27 and from then on, I have lived like this.

There is no information about his family of origin or his earlier life and identity, no recounting of how he met his wife or their marriage life beyond her illness and deterioration, no elaboration of his relations with her family, from whom he later bought the taxi business, no comment on the childhood or lives of his daughters, no mention of wider society – not even the Wende, which must have been particularly exciting for the private sector. It is as if the present has taken over the past and drawn a veil over the future; his life and his identity have become subsumed into his caring biography.

There is little opportunity for the marriage to build up routines, habits and emotional bonds prior to the onset of the disability. But for at least 18 years the fits are occasional, and Frau Speyer brings up the children and manages the household herself. Herr Speyer mentions in passing that his wife worked as a book-keeper, but she is attributed with no independent life or decision making, not even a partnership role in planning their life:

> Well, when we got married, I said, listen, I'd rather work an hour – I still was a lorry driver ... well I said, well you bring up the children and I bring in the money, that was my wish that my wife stayed at home.

In 1954 when they married, it was probably not unusual for women to opt for a housewife role. Women's employment was intensified after the building of the Berlin Wall in 1961 and the haemorrhaging of labour to the West. What is more unusual, spoken in the context of East Germany in 1992, is the representation of this decision as specifically his.

In depicting their marriage, which seems to go on relatively normally for many years, he highlights holidays and meals out that mark the road to the restriction of their lives. They are experiences of social embarrassment or when the limits of social acceptability are overstepped. There are many medical encounters, starting with the doctor's unfortunate advice to have another child: "What came with the child has to go with the child". In typical GDR style, Herr Speyer is sustained over the years by a particular woman doctor, who constantly advises the use of respite and residential provision. His narrative focuses on his steadfast refusal to use such services. The chief nurse from the social station, whom he likes, has persuaded him to accept nursing care for one hour a day, the maximum which can be provided free of charge:

> I was offered more help, well … I could have had help two or three times a day, but it wouldn't help me at all. I *have* to be there, because I can't leave her *alone*, she climbs out, bruised all over her body, because she will fall, she cannot walk.

It remains puzzling why Herr Speyer subsumes his identity into caring to such a degree, defying the norms of his sex and his society, making no reference to the costs of his actions to his taxi business (now run by his son-in-law), and separating himself off from social contacts and his family. While his strategy might be usual between spouses in the later stages of life, it certainly seems exceptional for a younger man.

Herr Speyer attributes his course of action to marital loyalty. He does not mention other possible reasons such as his dependency on his wife, his lack of social confidence, or the poor state of East German nursing homes for those who lacked party privileges[6]. As one of the social station nurses said, "I would never put my mother in such a place – not even my mother-in-law". Relations between Herr Speyer and his wife's family, with whom the couple live for the first four years of their marriage, could explain his strategy. Herr Speyer starts out as a lorry driver, and the circumstances under which he takes over the taxi business 18 years into the marriage, when Frau Speyer's condition is clearly deteriorating, are not explained. The taxi business certainly gives him more flexibility to look after his wife and family. What web of mutual obligations is involved can only be inferred.

By enhancing his heroism and sacrifice, he underplays the efforts and inputs of other people, such as his daughters. Before Frau Speyer's recent deterioration, the couple used to spend the winters in one daughter's flat, and the other daughter helps with heavy cleaning duties. However much more help there has been than he acknowledges, he seems determined to set himself apart from other people. His account resounds with pride, but when asked by the interviewer what he misses most, he responds with an emotional outburst at his loss:

> Overall in the last ten years, a bit of love. I had nothing. The drama was that I am no longer a man here, I am a woman, a housekeeper [three-second pause]. I had nothing that is normal in other marriages, where you get spoilt as a man a little bit, *nothing*. It's the other way around with us. Well, my life is up against a tree.

In the East German context, Herr Speyer's strategy of individualised self-sufficiency leaves him isolated. He seems unconnected with the informal networks which pervade East German society. His implicit intransigence seems to reflect the oppositional world of the private sector, constituted on the unspoken and unsayable values of the family's self-sufficiency and individualism. The patriarchal character of his self-presentation, which denies his wife any personality or pain of her own, is doubtless reinforced by the extent of her brain damage, but also emanates from an older era of family life[7].

Transition cases

Both the caring situations presented here are relatively new, and their accounts intertwine the new confrontation with disability with the collapse of the GDR. Reality and metaphor are interwoven as the external structure of the known society collapses inwards and the disability creates a restricted and encapsulating world. The decimation of the security, activity and sociability of employment is symbolised in the caring situation. Preoccupation with illness and disability may provide a refuge from the shock of events in the outside world, but it also prevents participation in a wider social process; unification offers new freedoms to which these carers are denied access. For 'transition' carers, the polarity between home and the outer world is extended and dramatised in a double tragedy, and they themselves 'switch' objectively and subjectively, in their attitudes and in their behaviour.

Unification brings a new emphasis on family responsibility in the welfare system, which adds to the 'family pull' which is inherent in a caring situation. Yet both women in the transition cases have the habit and expectation of a career outside the home, and their 'outward propulsion' serves them well in their search for services and supports. The family pull entails patriarchal processes, albeit different ones, since the two women are at opposite ends of their careers. The key struggle for Frau Blau (aged 60) is in the relationship with her husband, who has always taken the lead in presenting them as a couple in the public world. Taking command and experiencing marital power brings highly ambivalent feelings. For Frau Arndt (aged 23), accepting the support of her family, which she needs for her training, restores the dependencies of childhood and her father's patriarchal rule.

Immersion in their own troubles and pain blunts the awareness of both women to the feelings of those they care for. Frau Blau tends to infantilise and berate her husband, so that he suffers not just from his own incapacity but also from her furious frustration with him; Frau Arndt refers repeatedly to her son Claus as "annoying".

Frau Arndt

Frau Arndt is 20 when her son is born in December 1989, just at the time of the Wende. During the pregnancy, Frau Arndt's partner departs for the West. Frau Arndt's son has holes in his heart and is a Down's syndrome child. He communicates to a degree, though without speech, and is incontinent. Her enterprise having closed, Frau Arndt is now training in public employment, which will give long-term security. This necessitates living during the week with her parents and her grandmother in their small flat. Her father gets Claus up and takes him to the crèche in the morning, and Frau Arndt picks him up at four in the afternoon. Her mother helps her to deal with medical and social assistance appointments. She spends weekends in her own flat on an outlying estate, where she has a circle of friends and contact with other parents with disabled children. At the time of the second interview, she has completed her training, secured a daytime job, and moved back to her own flat. Her partner is around, but her family remain her main source of support and relief.

Frau Arndt describes Claus's birth as a time of "total crisis"; he is conceived in one social system and born into another. The interview takes place in her parents' flat, where she stays during the week. Her parents and Claus take part in the interview at times, and several times there is an interruption while Claus is attended to. The interview scenario portrays well the system of protective support in the family, together with its restrictions. Frau Arndt mostly speaks in a clipped style, scarcely mentioning her feelings, and focuses on present events, without discussion of her perspectives for her own life.

When the tape starts, the interviewer is assuring Frau Arndt that she can indicate at any time if she would like the recorder switched off. It seems that Frau Arndt has expressed a nervousness and vulnerability which has elicited special protection. Later on she admits that she has presented everything in a rather rosy and 'telegrammatic' style, which suggests an openness to being drawn into a more personal level of discourse. But her mother and father forestall that possibility by joining in, and the interview becomes increasingly interviewer-led. At the end, when Frau Arndt becomes upset and the interviewer switches off the recorder, they have a more personal discussion about her relationship with her partner and her "quite normal" life with Claus.

Frau Arndt and her parents portray themselves as victims of fate, incompetence, bureaucratic insensitivity and even deception. From the fortress of their family, the external world and the future look bleak and threatening. Frau Arndt's narrative begins with the birth, which she is told would be unproblematical. In fact, after two days of labour she is told it is a breech birth and given a Caesarean section. The baby is pronounced healthy, but three days later heart defects are identified. Frau Arndt's father spotted the abnormality. She is also infuriated by her interrogation by social assistance workers, and by the medical evaluation of Claus's level of disability, which determines the amount of care benefit. These experiences are invoked several times:

> Well as I said, one has so much trouble with the social assistance, with remarks like why didn't I want to go to work and so on, since the child can go to the crèche. So when the baby year was up, I still got that, the baby year, and they couldn't understand that at all, why such a young woman with a child doesn't want to go to work. And I say, I can't, he's got heart failure, I had him with me, "what's that, where is his heart failure?", and things like that, you're made out to be stupid [two-second pause]. Just so that you go to work as quickly as possible and don't cost them anything.
>
> They [the assessor] come for five minutes, look at the child, just as the last person did, the child looks fine. I say, believe me, that's a Down's

> child, nothing has changed, the doctors set him at 100% and that's it, isn't
> it. She couldn't quite grasp it, says "I've seen worse children". I say, well,
> grown-ups or other people also look different, you can't go by that. "Oh
> well, [two-second pause] we'll see." If she decides like that one will have
> to challenge it, but that means another fight.

Her father's account is a torrent of anger: "The problems just piled up at a stroke, that was what was so bad about the whole thing". He refers to the pregnancy, the disability, the father leaving, the firm going bust, the heart operation, the unemployment, the inadequate money, the threat of being a recipient of social assistance, the parents being liable, the run-around to find employment training, the crèche being too far from her work, his having to help in the mornings, the great-grandmother being there following illness which makes them a five-generation household (this is incorrect – they are a five-person, but four-generation household, living in three rooms) and the fact that "here you have to fight for every penny". The future is equally gloomy: the kindergarten is likely to be repossessed by the former owner, Frau Arndt will probably have to do shiftwork, violence against vulnerable people is increasing, pension and employment rights for disabled people have been removed, and the 'social state' is not at all caring.

Interpretation of the interview makes it clear that it is not Claus's disability as such which is 'the problem', but rather the pregnancy or perhaps the departure of Frau Arndt's husband. Silence reigns on these topics, yet they are inferred in the father's horror at the fate which, without his actions, might have befallen them collectively: "[after a pause] If they [Frau Arndt and Claus] hadn't had our help, that would have been a social case, one which would stay in the records [pause]". Thus the system of mutual family dependency is enforced not just by the material aspect of the West German system of intergenerational liability, but the moral aspect of impending shame which they would all have suffered. Frau Arndt's training in public employment is an investment for them all.

While Claus's disability heightens tensions in the family, he also keeps them together. Generally he is referred to by all of them as a nuisance and an object in the third person. The grandfather "puts Claus away" in the mornings, and his reappearance in the evenings causes conflict. Often it is impossible to say whether a sentence refers to him or to the general situation, and clearly the two are inextricable. This is exacerbated by the fact that in German the word for a child takes the neuter 'it' form. Frau Arndt's use of 'we' or of the impersonal 'one', which is more common in

German than in English, is also remarkable – she scarcely ever refers to herself in the 'I' form. The self-parody between Frau Arndt and her mother in the following comments makes the patriarchal structure of the family no less 'real':

Frau Arndt:	Well yes, when everyone comes home from work, everyone has something else, and then such a child [pause], one has a lot to do, either there's an explosion, or a real rumpus, but then it's good again [two-second pause]. That is not excluded, not that everything is always hunky-dory [two-second pause]. We subordinate ourselves, and grandfather always has the say with us.
Mother:	We all subordinate ourselves, all under grandad.
Frau Arndt:	Yes, that's true. We all have our feet under his table [laughter].

On the other hand, Claus binds the family together more positively. He insists that they all eat together, and in the summer they all go to Frau Arndt's garden because it makes him so happy if they all turn up. He also gives the great-grandmother a role in the family, because he loves her best, stroking her and listening to stories – he never bites her or bangs his head on the floor when he is with her.

Frau Arndt says her key problem is feeling so exhausted: "Giving attention [to Claus] and things to do, somewhere one is left behind". What is lost is her youth, her fun, her freedom for relationships – at least in the context of her family, for she talks quite differently about her life on her own estate. Here she is brighter, mentioning her own and Claus's enjoyments, depicting a situation in which she can be much more tolerant of his disruptions:

> ... yes ... we meet once a month, depending on how much time we have, and we're pleased when the children are together, and we can talk together. Now it's winter we all meet in the flat, and all three boys are lively [two-second pause] there's a real rumpus sometimes, but one can easily tolerate that [four-second pause].

She goes on to say how "out there" she knows lots of parents with children of Claus's age and experiences an ease with disability:

> No one says, "no we're not playing with that one", or anything like that, or "I'm not touching that one". Claus is treated like any other child. And that is really great, [three-second pause] it's really nice [four-second pause].

The family's representation of its situation contrasts strikingly with what has been achieved. Through their pressure, a well-known cardiologist performs the operation in good time, and Claus benefits early on from a physiotherapist and then a social worker. The social worker organises the parents group which still meets, which leads to Frau Arndt joining Lebenshilfe, a particularly active group concerned with mental disabilities. Through those connections, Claus joins an integrated crèche, and then a small kindergarten group with specialised staff. A Lebenshilfe lawyer appeals against the reduction of Claus's disability and benefit levels, Frau Arndt succeeds in getting alimony from her partner even though he claims he is unemployed, and now she has completed her training and got a daytime job. Claus is becoming more communicative and mobile, and at times she speaks of him with real pleasure – his enjoyment of the camping holiday with her sister, and the way he can make her roll about laughing, especially by his imitation of animal sounds. The family, which is relatively uneducated, seems to be saved from itself by the positive features of East German society, which continue after the Wende, and which give Frau Arndt both independence and support.

Frau Blau

> Frau Blau (aged 60) has just reached her office when she receives a phone call saying that her husband has had a stroke. He is almost completely paralysed. He is taken to hospital, but the flight of personnel to the West means that there are not even enough staff to do the bedpans. Once, Frau Blau finds him on the floor. At first she struggles to maintain her job. While the Wende has catapulted her husband, a transport engineer, into early retirement and then redundancy, she has been obliged to work full-time, and she values her improved pension prospects. Nevertheless, she soon decides to take him home, which entails an endless battle for services, equipment and benefits.

Two years on, exhausted and down two stone in weight, Frau Blau speaks of a process of personal change in which, as the couple's chief spokesperson, she is discovering an unnervingly forceful 'I'. Cajoled to make an effort and show enthusiasm for her plans for visits, sanitaria cures and disabled people's holidays, Herr Blau is gradually recovering some movement and speech. The couple have lost contact with work colleagues and their married daughter is preoccupied with her work. To their surprise, they have made friends with a gay couple next door. The Blaus have considered joining a disability group, but Herr Blau dislikes being identified with disabled people, and they both feel uncomfortable in a group of mainly younger people in wheelchairs.

In GDR days, Frau Blau worked as an administrator of supplies in a textile firm. She is used to daily contact with the outside world through her employment, Herr Blau's friends and colleagues, concerts and the opera. Their cupboard is full of books and brochures collected in preparation for travel in their retirement.

The loss of external contact makes them feel both confined and exposed. Frau Blau says: "Hmm [sighs], like in a bell-jar [pause]. Life goes on outside and we just watch [long pause]". Her succession of forays to various authorities is a means of maintaining outside contact, and her previous responsibility for supplies in GDR conditions doubtless gives her skills and persistence. Her narrative depicts Herculean struggles against authorities in the new system: for a phone, a lighter wheelchair, a bath lift, a better physiotherapist, pensions, care and holiday allowances, health cures. These accounts draw bitter analogies with the political privileges required for access to many services in the GDR. But while welfare services provide a conduit for access to the public sphere, Frau Blau feels guilty about leaving her husband, tending to rush back or telephone.

In order to get them out as a couple, she manoeuvres the wheelchair down the stairs for a walk round the block, and into the car for a visit to the garden, the market or the shops. She plans holidays and health cures, and a visit to relatives in West Germany. Herr Blau feels embarrassed by his disabled status, and Frau Blau resents his reluctance to brave the world. They both feel deprived of the advantages of unification, though they appreciate their new car and sound system.

At a more hidden level, Frau Blau's account suggests a family history of gendered conflicts around caring. Frau Blau's life encompasses extended caring, quite apart from her ongoing household responsibilities. Herr Blau loses his close family connections in his youth through death, remarriage and moves to the West, and Frau Blau herself belongs to a woman-centred family structure. Her mother cares for Frau Blau's daughter while Frau Blau is training professionally, and Frau Blau and her teenage daughter care intensively for her mother in her later years. Herr Blau is marginalised from this constellation and, following some unmentionable early incident between Herr Blau and his mother-in-law, she cannot live with them, even terminally. It may be that Frau Blau still feels resentful towards her husband about this – even that it causes her heart problems, as a result of which she works part-time for many years. Certainly caring as a family commitment is a structuring element in Frau Blau's biography, despite her ongoing outside career. But now the need for full-time care forces Frau Blau fully into the private sphere.

The shift to full-time care confronts Frau Blau with her own dependency within the marriage. If her struggle with the public sphere is one theme in her account, the other is her more private drama as an unappreciated wife, who has to carry the burden of care and now take the lead in the marriage relationship. These outer and inner dramas are connected, since her struggle with the welfare system shifts her position in the couple relationship. It is a separating experience for her, in which she risks losing her hold on partnership:

Frau Blau:	[pause] through this I have become much more independent, more independent than ...
Herr Blau:	You were like this before.
Frau Blau:	But not like this, Hans-Otto, I have to represent us completely to the outside world. Can I offer you some more [coffee]?
Interviewer:	No, thank you.
Frau Blau:	[pause] and I have to check myself sometimes, that I am not only speaking about myself, because I am out there alone, but that I am still [saying] 'we'...

While Frau Blau finds new personal strength in facing the world on her husband's behalf, it is difficult for her to separate herself out from the 'caring' aspect of her activities and from her husband. She is also afraid of her assertive and possibly vengeful sense of power and independence. Her view of the conflicts in their relationship become more explicit when the physiotherapist arrives and takes Herr Blau into the next room. Asked if she would accept an afternoon's or day's respite care she says:

> Yes, now yes. A year ago I said "no I won't do that, I don't want that", but today I see through that. Basically I don't get five minutes to myself. Sometimes I feel wiped out. He can't help it, but he's like a limpet, he takes me over completely and utterly. Before, we liked going to a concert, to the opera – that is all gone.

Clearly she is blaming her husband for her own susceptibility to feelings of dependency: "he takes me over completely". But perhaps neither partner can take on the perspective of the other. Herr Blau seems not to recognise the significance to Frau Blau of having to give up work just when she has begun to enjoy taking the economic lead in the household, or of the longstanding pattern of power in the marriage of which she is becoming newly aware. And she shows no empathy with his trauma of becoming disabled: her view is that if only he went out, things would be solved. That the conflict is lived out in a daily struggle for domination is painfully evident in the interview process, in which Frau Blau tries to prevent Herr Blau intervening in her lead role, and consistently infantilises him by criticising his contributions, which are minimal because of his speech difficulties.

Frau Blau is much more conscious of her dilemmas than Frau Arndt is, and more actively engaged in personal struggle. She has fewer support networks than Frau Arndt does, is fighting to change the dynamics of a long partnership, and faces the possibility of her husband having another stroke or not making much progress. Although Frau Arndt is less experienced and more passive, she has her own environment away from her family, and also has the future on her side. Claus is making claims on her which challenge her emotionally, and his progress through medical and educational institutions creates a learning experience. Objective developments will move Frau Arndt on, whereas Frau Blau's ability to combat domestic isolation will continue to rely on her strength of personality and the dynamic of her past experience.

Comparisons

We speculated that in East Germany caring might provide a refuge from the new competitive turmoil of the marketplace, in a context of high unemployment. It also seemed possible that caring might provide a counter-identity to the prescribed role of the emancipated employed woman under state socialism. Yet neither of these theories was borne out in any way. Nor did it seem the case that concern for economic security, including a future pension, and the desire to avoid the stigmatised status of being a 'social security case', were masking a deeper and more personal desire for an identity as a home carer.

Among the West German carers, although only Frau Jakob clings positively to an identity as a home carer, others quite easily tolerate the role, even if they appreciate some relief from it. Even Frau Hamann, who was previously a professional, does not really question her home-based role, only its extreme isolation. But in the case of East Germany, the carers show no such desire for a home-based identity or role; they are all determined to continue to develop or maintain their own professions and out-of-home identity. Even the most recent carers, who might be most susceptible to the Western-led pressures of unification, have a strong outward orientation.

From all the 26 original interviews in East Germany, only one person was prompted by caring to retreat into the private sphere. In so doing, rather than yielding to social pressures, Herr Speyer is defying both the official system and the informal culture of networking. Despite its exceptional nature, the case of Herr Speyer was useful in alerting us to the dimension of patriarchy in two other East German cases. Frau Arndt is involved in a struggle against the patriarchal regime of her father, which is certainly exacerbated by the new welfare system and its threat of stigmatising the whole family. Frau Blau is extricating herself from her dependency on her husband. But in neither of these transition cases is patriarchy the determining dynamic.

In East Germany, 'trawling the system' is the dominant dynamic, which the transition cases closely follow – it is the direction in which they are heading. Key factors in the East German pattern of outer-connectedness are work identities, the organisation of services outside the home and the culture of networking. A curious question, open to debate, is the extent to which these determining structural features can be attributed to intended policy.

We have already found a certain 'perversity' in the informal sector in West Germany in relation to formal policy – a cultural time lag in which family culture is retarded in comparison with policy developments, a bureaucratisation of welfare which contradicts the principles of subsidiarity, and a clash between individualised material incentives and more solidaristic ethical norms. We found that the formal features of the system as characterised in 'welfare regime models', which are weak in relation to the social services, are even weaker when applied to the informal sphere. The relatively large size of West German dwellings is an important facilitating factor in home care. Yet dwelling size is not included in welfare regime models, nor in most discussions of social policy. This illustrates the inevitable fuzziness of social policy boundaries.

Our East German cases likewise suggest a disjunction between formal and informal systems, although a key feature in East Germany was the absence of a policy on home caring. As indicated earlier, there was not even a word for caring and it was difficult to convey what our research was about. Nor were the strategies of carers lagging behind official policy – they were reaching outside and beyond it. The general tendency to outward-orientedness fully conforms with East German policy on women's employment and replacing and supporting family functions by collective services. The idea of maximising the capacities of disabled young people and giving them vocational training was also in line with the official system. But the means which the carers were using to achieve these goals lay outside or stretched official channels. Frau Meissner, the Grüns and Frau Arndt avoided the allocation of their children to certain institutions and gained access to others, invariably using the help of sympathetic professionals. Frau Blau's fight was to cut through red tape and speed up access to services and equipment. The fact that party control was focused on the workplace rather than community services seemed to allow more room for such discretionary action by professionals.

The use of informal networks was likewise part of the system, while not part of policy. In using networks to gain information and access to services, carers were simply using the everyday strategies of survival in East Germany, which had become a cultural form. The system of networks suited officialdom in that it substituted for its deficiencies, and remained sufficiently depoliticised to pose no obvious threat. As we have seen, the work collectives became the locus of a degree of counterculture as well as self-help. The slower pace and more relaxed attitude to work in East Germany meant that Frau Blau was able to extend her lunch hours to care for her mother. Katrin's school accommodated her mother, first as an odd-job person and then as school nurse. We used the phrase 'trawling the system' to suggest that carers were using what was there, but in doing so they hunted out services which were acceptable to them, using informal networks and personal determination to make their selection and gain access.

In supporting carers' avoidance of mainstream forms of institutional provision, sympathetic officials were of course acting in accordance with their professional values. As Anderson (1999) puts it, East German society was one in which "decent unpolitical lives could be led" and in which there was "some scope for residual idealism" (p 16). Such professional actions were expressive of the Lutheran and socialist humanism which pervaded East German culture, with which the ethic of mutual self-help was also aligned. Debates about how to characterise the East German regime have tended to emphasise its authoritarian and dictatorial nature. Jarausch (1998), reviewing these arguments, opts for the 'Fürsorgediktatur' (nanny dictatorship) as the term best able to combine the facets of authoritarianism and security in the GDR. Following Maier (1997), he argues that people settled for obedience in return for security, with a resultant "repression of independent initiatives in the private sphere". We return to these arguments in chapter five, but note here that whatever the effects at a more organised level of civil society, at the level of informal exchanges there was a most vigorous culture which, in a benign pattern of perversity, generated the very features of socialist cooperation which the political system seemed set to stifle.

The West German chapter's conclusion identifies the way in which new lines of social conflict and the influence of elites have blocked initiatives for reform and innovation arising at the margins of the Federal system (Vester, 1994). It suggests that innovative ideas from those who fall outside the traditional normative framework of caring do not filter through to the wider population, and that the disability movement in Germany has not penetrated mainstream political discourses in the way it has in Britain. The alternative milieus of the early 1980s were likewise marginalised by the main welfare organisations.

The interesting difference in the East German situation is that the main social system itself, shaped by everyday practices of survival and struggle, promoted for carers much of the dynamic which has only arisen at the margins of West German society. There was much more continuity between the practices of everyday life and the strategies of outward-oriented carers in East Germany than in West Germany. It is a tragedy that the speed of unification steamrollered the social infrastructures which generated such supportive forms of social exchange and engagement – although how they could have been grafted onto the market system is not obvious either. The loss and non-recognition of these valued structures may also lie at the heart of the bitterness to which commentators point. Pollack and Pickel (1998) argue that the key source of division between East and West Germany is cultural rather than economic, despite the persistence of material inequalities. The cultural sore lies in the dismissal of East German biographies and of East Germans as a 'social group', in an injuring of a sense of dignity and pride (p 22). Anderson likewise sees "a deep suppressed rage at the way the official version of the past dismisses as completely worthless the world of their childhood". He appeals for politics to be "in much closer touch with ways of life and feeling in the East" if an explosion is to be avoided (1999, p 16). Part of the value of our case studies of East German carers is that they allow a glimpse into some of the more positive aspects of this world which has now been lost.

Notes

[1] The difficulty of clarifying the terms 'caring' and 'carer' was even more difficult in East Germany than in West Germany, so that identifying who we wanted to speak to – in letters and phone calls and even in face-to-face situations – was a real problem. Since the clients of staff in the social stations were the disabled people, and given the lack of direct prior communication with the interviewees (few telephones) it was quite difficult to resist being 'given' disabled interviewees rather than carers. In one case, the carer was disabled. As a consequence, we conducted several additional interviews with disabled people, which extended our knowledge of disability in East Germany.

[2] In general, the interviewees warmed to the fact that the study was for a 'lady from London', especially one who had conducted research in East Germany before and knew it quite well. This seemed to be the case whether the interviews were conducted by the 'lady' herself or by local interviewers.

[3] Through extensions to maternity leave, delivered with considerable fanfare at the party conference each year, 'the baby year' had reached three years by the late 1980s, causing problems in workforce management. Crèche and kindergarten provision was fully available, although not in the proximity of 600 metres from home, which had been promised.

[4] There were sharp conflicts among local leaders as to what 'participation' should consist of: for 'reform communists', socialism required the mobilisation of independent rights and interests; for the 'new guard', local anger was a spur to efficiency; for the 'old guard', it was an opportunity to explain difficulties and win patience and loyalty from the population (Chamberlayne, 1990a, pp 157-8).

[5] Fear of going out alone meant that elderly people needed to be accompanied by Zivis or home helps to go shopping or for a walk. Fear of assault and burglary was commonly mentioned in the interviews with carers, and seemed to express

the general sense of precariousness and invasion which the 'Wende' brought. The media gave great prominence to thefts and muggings.

[6] Nursing homes provided a hierarchy of conditions, with single rooms for party members and war veterans who had taken a stance against Nazism.

[7] For the strength of traditional gender relations in the informal sphere in Eastern Europe, see Watson (1993) and Dölling (1995). In this view, traditional gender relations were sustained far beyond the private sector.

FOUR

Britain – sitting on the doorstep

Introduction

Our characterisation of British informal caring as 'sitting on the doorstep' indicates a pattern of care in which the private, public and social spheres of welfare interact to produce highly individualised and precarious caring strategies.

Common to the experiences of carers in Britain is that their caring strategies shift around within the support triangle of family, the social sphere and formal services, depending on changing circumstances and needs. While the home and family remain central to their experiences, the private, social and public spheres of care appear less separate and mutually exclusive to the lives of carers than in the German societies. Carers in Britain typically combine care, employment and wider voluntary and social activity, and care is shared with partners.

This chapter begins with a discussion of the welfare context of informal care in Britain, drawing on social policy debates around informal welfare, and discussing the impact of the recent community care legislation at national and local levels. The case studies are presented in the second section, introducing the three British categories of carer strategies. In the third section, we discuss the cases in the light of salient themes in the British welfare context and consider comparisons with the two German contexts.

Formal and informal welfare in Britain

The cultural basis of welfare

The British welfare state is embedded in a long and influential tradition of liberalism, which espouses a notion of freedom through individual responsibility and the limitation of state provision (Esping-Anderson, 1990; Chamberlayne, 1999). This philosophy, returned to under Margaret Thatcher, has formed an ideological counterpoint to the postwar welfare state ideals of equality and citizenship, which informed many of the developments in welfare between 1945 and 1979 (Douglas and Philpott, 1998).

Freeman and Rustin (1999) argue that these two traditions in welfare form the dual anchoring of the British welfare system. They are expressed in the coexistence of collectivist values of equality of opportunity and provision through the welfare state, and the liberal individualist values of private education and home ownership, for example, as well as in the personal enhancement of life chances through market mechanisms (p 9). As a result, British social policy developments are characterised by contradictory policies, which shift between universalist aspirations (as realised, for example, in child benefit payments) and selective, means-tested provision according to need (many of the social security policies) (Hartley, 1994).

The duality of the welfare norms of individualism and state provision is not simply an important point of reference for policy makers and welfare providers; this duality is often shared by those receiving welfare. Baldock (1998) cites the example of the system of direct, free or subsidised local authority service provision for older people, used until the late 1980s:

> People and their families would help themselves as much and for as long as they could. Pure technical entitlements were not necessarily taken up. Yet when an older person's family and private support broke down, or when the 'risks' seemed too high, state help was given to some degree outside strict measures of need or ability to pay. It was a bootstrap system built on shared values as to state and citizen's obligations and entitlements. (p 167)

Administratively confused and disorganised, direct provision was regulated by a shared cultural understanding between professionals and the public about who could be helped and when. Given this background, it may be less surprising that the welfare state developed as the main provider of social welfare, in contrast to the continental traditions of tripartite (individual, community and state) welfare structures. While the system as such remained residual and inconsistent, it provided continuity in terms of a shared understanding that state assistance would be available, if the need should arise.

The 1970s brought forward new and competing perspectives and values to different social arenas. The change was also the consequence of a fiscal crisis of the state, resulting in an era of sustained stagnation and reduction in public expenditure (Freeman and Rustin, 1999; Douglas and Philpott, 1998). Thatcherite and post-Thatcherite neo-liberal ideas gave a new impetus to the notions of individual responsibility and self-sufficiency in meeting personal welfare needs (Le Grand and Bartlett, 1993; Baldock, 1998). These ideas were played out in the numerous discussions around public and private responsibilities for welfare, the role of the family and, most importantly, in debates around the 'proper' relationship between welfare needs and service provision. Coupled with a drive for a rationalised 'governance' of social policy, the Conservative agenda included the restructuring of social policy arenas according to the values of 'efficiency, effectiveness and economy' and remoulded institutions of public bureaucracy according to the values of private sector 'managerialism', market approaches and the emerging 'institutional economics' (Bochel and Bochel, 1998; Le Grand and Bartlett, 1993; Lewis and Glennerster 1998).

The introduction of the community care legislation in 1990 can be seen as a major departure from the collective, state-centred system of welfare provision (Deakin, 1994). Walker (1994) distinguishes four areas of structural change in local formal welfare provision through the community care legislation: 1) the fragmentation of social services, local decision making and implementation; 2) a privatisation of services; 3) marketisation through the introduction of contracts for a variety of services and the purchasing role of local authorities; and 4) rationing by limiting resources available through the contracts.

Guided by ever-reducing service budgets, criteria of eligibility and entitlements have become the lynchpin in making decisions about service provision. Services are only free to those who fall within the boundaries of locally fixed eligibility criteria. For those who fall outside these criteria, or who require additional services not covered, self-payment is the only alternative.

Organisationally, the legislation has shifted the provision of public welfare into a 'community' context, in the form of community-based projects and approaches and, most often, through a system of support in the home and through family. Intellectually, it has reaffirmed the expectation that individuals and families should provide care for 'their own'. As publicly provided services are reduced, 'privatised' or provided by voluntary organisations, renewed emphasis is placed on family responsibility and "personal ties of kinship, friendship and neighbourhood" (Lewis, 1993, p 4). This has consequences for the structure of welfare services, but has also had an impact on the political struggle for entitlements and the recognition of welfare needs.

There are few indications that there has been a fundamental departure from these principles in the development of community care under the Labour government in the latter part of the 1990s. While recent legislation stresses a partnership model among state agencies, voluntary organisations and the private sector, moving away from the market model, the emphasis remains on individual responsibility (Department of Health, 1998). For example, the Royal Commission on Long-term Care (1999) stresses in its findings the "shared responsibility of individual and state" in preparing for and providing long-term care.

Informal welfare

Social policy commentators such as Jane Lewis and Peter Taylor-Gooby argue that the divisions between formal and informal spheres of welfare and between paid and unpaid work became more pronounced during the 1980s and early 1990s, as a consequence of the Conservative agenda for welfare (Lewis, 1993, p 4; Taylor-Gooby, 1991). Taylor-Gooby estimates that the contribution of unpaid work in Britain amounted to £24 billion in wage equivalence in 1990 (Taylor-Gooby, 1991, pp 100-1). In 1994, there were around 7 million informal carers in Britain (Douglas and Philpott, 1998, p 136).

Women, in particular, have been affected by policy shifts towards family-based welfare, as they continue to carry much of the now increased unpaid work in the home (Kofman and Sales, 1996; Langan and Ostner, 1991, p 131; Lewis, 1993, p 5; Bennington and Taylor, 1993). As women's participation in the labour market is growing markedly, it leaves them in the position of having to balance both spheres of work, intensifying the burden of care responsibility and care labour. British feminists have argued that this has been one of the reasons for the continued inequality of women in employment. In Britain, women have remained trapped in the most insecure segments of the labour market, characterised by short, part-time work contracts, and low working hours and earnings: in 1990, 43.7% of women worked in part-time manual jobs, and 31.8% worked in non-manual jobs less than 16 hours a week (Lewis, 1993, p 10). This pattern of work has excluded a significant proportion of women from access to welfare benefit thresholds. With the change of government in 1997, the policy agenda has shifted to some extent. Current initiatives on pre-school, childcare and social security arrangements for informal carers are aimed at redressing the gender imbalance. These measures are limited, but they are certainly a step in the right direction.

Community care

The restructuring of personal welfare services from 1993 onwards through implementation of the community care legislation affected a number of aspects of service provision. It ended the institutionalisation of care for the most dependent groups: older people, people with disabilities and people suffering from mental illness. The most visible sign of this renewed community emphasis has been the closure of large long-term institutions over the last decade, both National Health Service (NHS) institutions and local authority residential homes, a move in which patients were either transferred to private or voluntary sector accommodation or rehomed within community settings (Peace et al, 1997; Department of Health, 1997). The policy emphasis for these vulnerable groups is shifted to the 'community', through a service combination of informal, voluntary, private and public provision.

While the pace of change varies in different areas of the country, the aspirations of the legislation have been to integrate these hitherto marginalised groups into a wider social setting. For older people, for example, the policy has shifted away from the approach of 'institutional neglect' (intervention as an emergency measure) of their care needs, towards a much more proactive approach of home-based support, dependency prevention and the recognition of individual needs (Douglas and Philpott, 1998, p 97). Professionals and clients have welcomed this aspect of the legislation.

The introduction of eligibility criteria for free services, specific funding arrangements on an individual basis, care packages and new organisational structures for case management have led to a more individualised approach in assessing care needs. Decisions about eligibility are made transparent through repeated care assessments, which recognise and record current and future requirements. Assessment is also a planning tool for local authorities and social services for developing community care strategies in the local community, in the form of community care plans, in which social services set out detailed service development plans for community care (Lewis and Glennerster, 1998)[1].

Community care has also changed the role of social services and social work itself. As social services have taken on the role of service planners rather than providers, the emphasis of the work has shifted towards local strategic development and financial and service management (Hoyes and Means, 1993). In the 'mixed economy of care', which incorporates a range of public, private and voluntary care providers, local authorities and social services have the role of purchasers and enablers of care services, emphasising the managerial role of social services as a statutory agency rather than any provider function (Le Grand and Bartlett, 1993).

The role of social work professionals has also changed considerably. They are increasingly taking up the role of managers who organise support services for clients, supervising frontline staff, instigating need assessments and controlling care budgets. Professionally, the 'social work' aspect of their role, in the form of person-centred work, community development and facilitation, is increasingly being replaced with that of a social administrator (Douglas and Philpott, 1998, p180 ff; Banks, 1995; Timms, 1983). For example, the introduction of care manager posts as intermediary professional positions between clients and social workers poses questions as to what type and quality of support clients can expect from frontline social services.

What have been the effects of the changes outlined above for informal care?

As local social services budgets remain subject to financial restrictions, many of the community social care services have been subject to repeated cuts and reductions, despite increasing demand for services. Direct support services, such as home-help schemes, have been reduced substantially in some areas. The gaps left have been only partially filled by the growing numbers of voluntary and private service providers operating in local areas. These are already the main providers of 'softer' support services, for instance in the form of carer support centres and telephone helplines (Douglas and Philpott, 1998, p 103). Changes in other areas, for example the reduction of NHS long-term beds in many localities, have added to the pressures locally.

Baldock (1999) argues that the changes have contributed to a climate of insecurity, particularly for older people, whose expectations about the welfare system do not correspond to the values of care management and self-reliance. In their research with stroke patients, Baldock and Ungerson (1994) found that for many older people, the experience of need and financial assessments, the range of alternative service options and the changing 'rules' of the formal care system are deeply disturbing and unsettling. For professionals and clients alike, community care has fundamentally changed the cultural underpinning of state-provided social services.

In the cases we studied, a common thread across their subjective experience is that community care policy has only had a limited positive impact on their lives. While most of the carers we interviewed had social services contact and had received some form of assessment, improvements in provision had been marginal and the social services were regarded as remote. Indeed, most of the carers had experienced some form of service change or reduction in recent years and certainly knew about service changes in their area. For some of the longstanding carers, the offers of additional or new services had been unacceptable because they were felt to interfere too much with their particular lifestyles.

Voluntary organisations, disability groups and carer groups

The role of voluntary organisations and that of private providers in the mixed economy of care has been increased (Lewis and Glennerster, 1998, p 7). Voluntary organisations at a local level have always fulfilled provider functions, such as meals-on-wheels services provided through agencies like Age Concern, or children's homes run by Barnardo's. After the introduction of the community care legislation, voluntary organisations found themselves increasingly in a formalised contractual relationship with local authorities to provide segments of services in line with mainstream service provision. For Means and Smith (1994), this constitutes a major cultural shift for local authorities and voluntary agencies alike.

The dilemma posed for local voluntary organisations is how to find an appropriate balance between increasing partnership and potential contractual subordination by state institutions, and the need to retain a more radical outlook as independent and decentralised spaces for social community-based action. Many of the voluntary agencies developed since the 1970s have worked specifically for the interests of otherwise neglected groups in communities, addressing some of the demographic deficits and inequalities in areas such as access to services, advocacy and community representation, often in difficult financial circumstances and on a small-scale basis (Kendall and Knapp, 1997, p 266). With voluntary organisations being pulled into the mainstream of the mixed economy of care, there are concerns that individual agencies will lose vital aspects of their independence and freedom, and that collectively the local landscape of community groups will suffer as some groups are favoured over others, leaving the rest to survive on reduced resources, unrecognised and neglected (Kendall and Knapp, 1997, p 267).

A comparable dilemma is apparent in the contrasting ways in which the carers movement and the disability movement have reacted to government reform and local implementation of community care policy. While the former seems to have entered into close partnership with social services, user groups for disabled people have maintained greater distance from the formal welfare agencies. As social services are recast as enablers of local service provision and clients become service users, contested arenas for user activism have emerged around concepts such as 'user empowerment', 'user involvement' and 'user participation' (Douglas and Philpott, 1998, p 140). While 'user empowerment' shifts power from the professional to the user, challenging the hierarchies of authority and influence, 'user involvement' is a less precise term which describes different modes of user participation in service policy and planning (Philpott, 1994).

Literature on empowerment tends to be centred on a discourse of individual rights rather than one of social relationships, although it may well emphasise the political importance of collective solidarities. Many writers argue that the carers' movement has been colonised or incorporated, and that 'consumer power' among carers amounts to consultation rather than participation (Barnes and Walker, 1996; Gordon and Donald, 1993). Barnes (1997) regrets that carer groups have formed an alliance with professional decision makers rather than with the more independent and militant disability groups, whereas others argue that a powerful combination of forces supports the emphasis on empowerment and that there is a need for training in participation among both professionals and users (Braye and Preston-Shoot, 1995; Smith et al, 1993). Barnes (1997) appreciates the advantages of information, trust and partnerships formed with the professional world, and Phillips (1996) likewise welcomes the developing of new skills of advocacy and negotiation which care planning entails, and the more open visibility of the tension between commitment and self-interest in caring situations. On the other hand, Clarke (1996) argues that the 'cultural revolution' of mission statements, corporate culture and quality review, together with struggles over power and instability, produce inward-looking services. As a consequence, research tends to focus on forms of organisation among professionals rather than on the interface with clients.

Nationally, the carers movement found recognition in the 1996 Carers (Recognition and Services) Act, which provides the right for a separate needs assessment for informal carers. Carers' organisations are now an accepted voice in local communities, although their influence in local service planning seems to be limited (see for example Glendinning and Bewley, 1992; Holzhausen, 1997). However, the two boroughs in our study (see below) have very active carer groups, which have developed into important resource and information centres for otherwise often isolated informal carers.

In contrast, disability groups have contributed significantly to the politicisation of welfare subjects, sponsoring a proactive 'struggle' for welfare rights based on the notion that disability is socially constructed, through discrimination and lack of access to social and cultural resources (Oliver, 1994; Barnes et al, 1999). The political philosophy of disability groups often results in tense relationships with social services and local authorities. Political activism on disability has provided a focal point of struggle against shortcomings and grievances, pushing government bodies to re-examine the basis of entitlements and service provision. Nationally, the campaign for direct payments, which resulted in the 1996 Community Care (Direct Payments Act), enables disabled people to purchase their own services.

Local community care

The two boroughs in London from which our British cases are drawn implemented the community care guidelines differently, demonstrating that despite the central directives of policy planning, care management strategies and various partnership agendas with voluntary agencies, community care at the local level involves the local interpretation of service needs and approaches.

East London borough

The East London borough is an ethnically and culturally diverse inner-city area of London. Some 44% of its residents are from ethnic minorities (1991 census), with the Indian community representing the largest minority ethnic group (13%). The borough is characterised by a high level of poverty and social deprivation. In 1992, 55% of households were in the low income bracket (income below £10,000 per annum). The degree of unemployment, particularly among some of the minority ethnic groups, is above the national average. A specific problem in this borough is the poor quality of the housing stock, much of which is substandard and lacks basic amenities. There is a substantial degree of overcrowding in some areas. Other indicators of social deprivation include above-average mortality rates for all age groups, and high levels of morbidity and long-term illness. There have been longstanding problems with health service provision, in particular community and child healthcare services, which have affected cooperation between health and social care services and which have posed problems for service coordination across agencies, although the 1997-2002 community care plan shows increased partnership working initiatives and liaison work.

Politically, the East London borough is a traditional Labour borough, with a long history of a vigorous multiethnic approach in local government planning. In 1991, it adopted a politically high-profile approach to its community care plan. One central plank in the development of its community care policy was to work through consultative and partnership initiatives with different ethnic groups, statutory groups, and specialist task and pressure groups, such as the HIV/AIDS organisation and older people's groups, towards a pluralist framework for community care development. Particular emphasis was placed on cooperation with the local community, and voluntary groups were seen as essential in gaining access to user and client groups and making their needs visible.

The local authorities had considerable success in attracting the support of some of the more mainstream organisations, such as the local carers' forum and some of the larger charities. More recently, in line with the 1997-2002 community care plan, the borough has created a number of posts to support carers. For example, outreach workers target carers from ethnic minorities and young carers.

Despite these initiatives, developing a multicultural approach to community care has been difficult. In 1993, a survey commissioned by the social services on the needs of ethnic community groups found profound distrust of, and disillusionment with, the local authorities' community care approach and policies among ethnic community groups. Provision offered under the community care arrangements was perceived to be of poor quality, under-resourced and racist in that it was marginalising and unresponsive to the needs of minority ethnic groups (Focus Consultancy Ltd, 1993). The community care strategy could not, for example, address the severe shortage of residential accommodation, transport needs and ethnically sensitive domiciliary services for its Afro/Caribbean and Asian communities. Moreover, a number of the small longstanding ethnic community care projects felt sidelined by the new community care approach, and under-resourced.

North London borough

The North London borough is largely middle class and, despite some pockets of deprivation, affluent. The borough adopted a cautious approach to community care after 1991. The initial community care plan targeted domiciliary services for the older population, with an explicit intention to maintain older people in their own homes. It also began to use mainly mainstream and established voluntary and private service providers.

Around 70% of the housing is owner occupied, with a large older population, particularly in the 75+ age range (1991 census). Some 20% of the population come from minority ethnic groups, among them long-established and affluent Jewish and Asian communities with flourishing community lives. The borough has a long tradition of community and self-help groups, which originally emerged as part of the community movements in the 1960s and 1970s.

The area is served by two district hospitals and a series of community health facilities. According to the 1995-96 community care plan, the largest group of users of social services are aged 85 and over, with 81% referred for social services assessment. Proposed developments under the community care plan include increases in disability support services, for example in the form of holiday schemes and a limited number of day-care facilities, and the promotion of specialist care for clients and carers from ethnic minorities, as well as the development of a consultative committee for carers.

In the late 1990s, areas of conflict with local pressure groups and representative groups of service users have emerged over the continued provision of facilities for health and social care services, such as long-term hospital places, respite facilities and community health facilities, which have been cut and sidelined through the increasing emphasis on domiciliary services. Carer groups, disability groups and pensioners groups, in particular, feel that they are losing out on such vital back-up services.

The North London borough has a thriving tradition of voluntary organisations and support groups among ethnic and cultural groups, which have worked independently for the benefit of their communities. Organisations such as Jewish Care continue to remain a focal point for care provision for the Jewish community, for example. Similarly, support groups and campaign groups have a long tradition in the locality, supported through comparative affluence. Although some efforts have been made to integrate them further into the care provision, in the 1994-95 community care plan they had not been systematically included into an overall care strategy. Indeed, some of the voluntary organisations involved in care service provision and support were intent on retaining their independence and respective community profiles.

The experience of both boroughs in implementing community care highlights Walker's argument that, because of the constraints of structural changes imposed on local councils in the community care legislation, the aspirations for local community care cannot be fulfilled (Walker, 1994, p 204). The East London borough, hampered by funding restrictions in local authority budgets, has difficulties in responding to the needs of the most deprived communities. In the North London borough, structural changes in other areas, such as the health services, contribute to the reduction in particular service areas, setting the authority on a collision course with local voluntary agencies. Both boroughs increasingly also need to target services on a smaller number of priority areas and a smaller group of clients.

In subsequent planning cycles, the discrepancy between the theory and reality of community care seems to have taken this gap into account by providing a detailed breakdown of progress in clearly identified target areas, with costed plans for further developments. The plans include partnership initiatives with other statutory providers, such as health services, delineating in quite precise terms what can be achieved within the given time period. While the expectations of service delivery have risen, the realities of community care fall short of them.

Carer strategies

Following this characterisation of the British welfare context, we distinguish three approaches to informal caring which structure caring over and above the contingencies of the physical aspect of the dependency, approaches which are influenced by emotional and intra-familial dynamics of caring.

In the first category, 'creating the social', carers actively embrace caring as a source of a new social identity and a pathway to action. The two carers in this group are both men, who find meaning and support in participating in new social networks. Carers in the second group, 'family is best', find at least a temporary solution to the pressures of changing circumstances by looking back to their families for support and assistance. A third group of carers, 'reluctant transitions', emerge tentatively from previously family-centred caring strategies. Their transitions result from personal crisis and often involve a painful process of reorientation.

Creating the social

Carers in this group have developed a proactive way of living with their caring responsibilities. Mr Allahm, a church founder, and Mr Merton, an activist for welfare and disability rights, are very different in terms of background and detail. However, their identities and everyday lives as carers are bound up with an active engagement in their local community. They participate in local disability and carer groups, bringing a public dimension to their informal caring activity. Their social identity as carers transcends the confinement of caring in the private sphere.

In developing these outward-oriented caring strategies, these male carers do not undergo the tumultuous and difficult processes of personal transitions or traumatic experiences that some of the East and West German carers undergo. They can tap into an already existing active social sphere, which is welcoming and receptive to their particular needs.

Mr Allahm

North London borough

Mr Allahm is 65 and cares for his wife (64). The Allahms originally came from Sri Lanka and had a varied life in different countries. Shortly after Mr Allahm's retirement, his wife shows symptoms of progressive dementia, which leave her increasingly confused and incapacitated. Mr Allahm is the main carer to his wife; he buys in professional help when required. His life revolves around his wife and around a church group, which he helped to found in response to the lack of spiritual support for people like himself.

Mr Allahm is a retired chemist, born in Sri Lanka, who has a senior career as a United Nations (UN) employee and later as a civil servant in Britain. He works extensively in Africa, leading a cosmopolitan lifestyle in the expatriate communities of the different nations he serves. As a young couple, Mr and Mrs Allahm become estranged from their Sri Lankan families and have to leave the country, because their love marriage violates the cultural traditions of Sri Lankan society at the time. Although they never settle back in their home country, eventually they re-establish links with their families.

The Allahms lead a traditional family life. Mr Allahm is preoccupied with his career, while Mrs Allahm is the homemaker and the centre of the family. Their four children are brought up in boarding schools in Britain, as the family have to move frequently with different UN postings. It is Mrs Allahm who remains the anchor point in the family's life. Mr Allahm's relationship with his children has never been particularly close: "She was the kingpin of the family, I hardly did anything; I was involved in my work...."

One of the strategies the couple use to counteract the many changes and transience of their different postings is to participate actively in the expatriate communities, especially in church activities. Mr Allahm, in particular, is an active and devoted church member wherever his career takes him: "my side activity was my church work ... so whatever time I had, I did work in connection with [that]...."

The family eventually settle in Britain permanently, and Mr Allahm works as a civil servant until his retirement in the late 1980s. Shortly after her husband's retirement, Mrs Allahm becomes increasingly frail. She is eventually diagnosed with dementia. She deteriorates rapidly, and is fully dependent on 24-hour care. The couple are financially well off, and Mr Allahm can buy in domestic help and carework assistance.

The most difficult aspect of caring for Mr Allahm is living with his wife's diminishing personhood. She does not recognise him, herself, or her surroundings. He and his wife have led a very close married life and have hardly been separated during their marriage. They have made their relationship the centre of their existence. With her progressing dementia, his personal anchor point to his life is gone and his love has died:

> We had lots of plans after I retired...my wife was a very active person and my wife was keen on doing a world tour ... it is not those that we miss, you see, rather, I don't have her as I knew her and ... I don't know what exactly goes through her mind.

The anguish this causes him emerges in his wish for family support, which was customary in Sri Lankan culture during his youth.

> In our culture, people don't stop to think how they have made it, it's because somebody helped you as a child ... mother, father and other people, grandfather, gran....

His own children lead their own professional lives and so cannot share in the day-to-day care of their mother. His three daughters, for example, all work and have small children, a fact which continues to cause intergenerational debate in the family. While he accepts that his own children have been brought up by different cultural values, he still wishes it were different:

> It was not our thing to get a wife to work and make money, you should provide for the wife. I was wrong, I was a male chauvinist, that's what they call them now [laughs] but that was our culture you see, I accept that, I accept it. The children ought to know, but in fact I tell them: "You shouldn't be working, you should be bringing up the children".

Mr Allahm receives help and advice from the carer organisation, and other local contacts. His church contact becomes a substitute for extended family support. He also co-founds a local group, in which members support each other spiritually and practically:

> I used to take my old ladies to get their toenails cut and ... it was very rewarding work, you know, when one old lady said ... thank you so much.... I did this work and things like that, now that my turn has come I am on the receiving end.

Other church members support him in practical aspects of caring for his wife, by occasionally cooking for him or doing his laundry.

The strategy of immersing himself in the church community makes the increasing stress of caring for his ailing wife bearable. He is involved in the different aspects of the church and also attends other carer groups and neighbourhood groups. In these activities he finds affirmation as a carer. He is able to give meaning to his current life by a framework of religious devotion and belief:

> I am sorry if I bore you by keeping on about faith, but that's the only thing that keeps us sane in this matter. Life has more meaning ... I accept this cross willingly. It is what we are called to do, that is my vocation to look after this lady and make the evening of her life something she will sort of not regret too much.

Lately, however, as his wife's dementia worsens and her dependency increases, the circumstances at home become progressively restrictive. Mr

Allahm has less time for his social life and voluntary activities, despite the fact that he has care services throughout the week. This does not suit his outgoing personality and lifestyle, and he feels increasingly restricted. His children are pushing him to seriously consider residential or nursing care for their mother. He is reluctant to agree to this:

> No, no not now, not now. Not if we can get someone to, I don't know, it looks as though, see it is not for us to decide, you see, care time might come. I don't know, if she becomes completely vegetable I don't know what, but our options now are to keep at home so that I may be with her and make her feel...

As a way out of his current dilemma, Mr Allahm is resorting to his own family ties in Sri Lanka, which he and his wife left behind so many years ago. His retired sister-in-law from Sri Lanka has suggested moving to Britain to become a live-in carer and companion to his wife, in effect sharing in the increasing demands of care and continuing the care for his wife:

> I've had a letter from my wife's sister in Sri Lanka – she is single and she is a teacher – she says ... she wants to give it all up and wants to come to look after her. The problem is, you know, what the visa implications are, so I'm going to consult on that and also a few other things for closing up the house there and things like that.

Mr Merton

East London borough

Mr Merton is in his forties. He is the main carer to his wife, who is in her thirties. Both are registered disabled and describe their arrangement as 'caring for each other'. Mrs Merton requires greater assistance in her daily life and uses a wheelchair intermittently. The couple are well-known disability campaigners in their local area and give advice on how to negotiate with authorities over benefits and services. In addition, Mr Merton also provides assistance to a number of older people in the neighbourhood.

Mr Merton's personal experience of ill health and disability is the result of epilepsy developed in his twenties. He comes from an East End working-class family. Shortly after leaving school, he joins the merchant navy for a number of years. When he returns home, he drifts from job to job. His most constant occupation is that of lifeguard in local swimming pools, a job he enjoys because of the athleticism and physicality involved:

> I worked for...for six months and then I went to sea, with the merchant navy. And then I came back and started...I'd done a bit of lifeguard work [before] and when I came back I continued doing lifeguard work ... If I tried to remember every single job I had it would be mind-boggling.

His various attempts at different jobs also include a temporary job as a care assistant working with disabled children. Retrospectively, this and his work as a lifeguard are episodes in his life which connect his past and current life as a carer:

> I've never had difficulty in caring. I used to look after disabled children and people in the swimming pool as a lifeguard, so I've always been a bit of a carer [laughs].

> I can jump into a situation very quick and I just get on with it. I mean, looking after someone for me is [five-second pause] I suppose very easy. Always done it. I've done it when I was younger.

His personal life is equally non-committed and fluid. He drifts from one relationship to another, marries once, but soon divorces. He has three children by different women, but only maintains contact with one.

His life turns with the onset of his own health problems. He has a series of epileptic fits, which need to be controlled by medication and which cut his working life short.

He has to stay in hospital for prolonged periods of time to stabilise his condition. He meets his wife in a residential hospital outside London. She has also developed severe epilepsy in her adulthood and has been an intermittent wheelchair user since her early twenties.

> Well, we just met in the hospital in C.... And we met there and I dealt with Kerry's fit in there [laughing], while the nurses were coming in ... Kerry and I made friends and in the end I said "Well I'll come and visit you every week, and if you come out, if you need to have somewhere to live, I've got a flat" and we just got on from there really.

The couple marry and live in East London borough. He is now the main carer for his wife, who cannot be left alone for long because of her epilepsy. In recent years, he also begins to support his elderly mother, who lives close by. Through his marriage, Mr Merton is introduced to disability rights issues through Mrs Merton's campaigning work, and is now an active member of different groups in the community and a respected local campaigner. Over the years, he develops a role as an advisor and advocate for local disabled and older people, checking in on them, carrying out errands and so forth, and also providing some personal care:

> If one of the elderly was to phone up, or one of the other disabled, we'd be down there ... and I'd try to do what I could. I mean, we had an old lady here the other year, who died. Lovely, and I used to go down and change the [incontinence] bag on her legs.

Mr Merton's experience of personal disability and informal care provides him with a focus to his life, which has previously been lacking. 'Campaigner' is a full-time occupation for him, and a focus of action which encompasses all aspects of his life:

> Twenty years ago, people like us would have been locked up.... Britain is a slow-moving country compared with others.... We don't want different treatment except that they recognise that she is using her wheels as her legs.

The expression 'people like us' signifies also a new identity as a disabled person, an identity he shares with his wife, forming the basis of their mutually supportive relationship. This closeness in perspective and bond is apparent in the interviews, which were in part conducted with the couple. The couple often take turns in narrating aspects of their life, each of them picking up the thread from the other, completing stories for each other without deviation or contradiction:

> Mrs Merton: What happened was that the doctors said that my legs collapsing was a psychosomatic condition. And to say that something is psychosomatic is bad.
>
> Interviewer: Are there no specialists then?

Mr Merton:	It is too expensive to go and see the only specialist in the country.
Mrs Merton:	It must be something in the water to only happen to people in the north or the west country [laughs].
Mr Merton:	London doctors try to find out about it as much as possible, but....

For Mr Merton, being a husband, caring for his wife, campaigning and his voluntary activities are all important elements in adjusting to a new life after his illness, and in staving off the debilitating effects of his own disability. As a strategy of personal adaptation, it is a very successful way of dealing with and coming to terms with a severe crisis in his life, brought on by his illness. Mr Merton does not look back on his former life with great regret – he values his present life as meaningful and rewarding. He has been able to leave behind his former rather isolated and isolating existence and build a life within his local community:

I mean, I think a lot of Kerry [his wife]. I mean, Kerry knows that if there's something wrong, I'd know, even if she didn't, I would.... It's satisfying to know [five-second pause] I suppose I had a bit of a hard life [three-second pause] Kerry had a bit of a hard life and I suppose ... it's just come to a conclusion that we're both fairly well-suited. We're fairly well-suited and she knows how to deal with my fits and I know how to deal with her illness. [His wife laughs.]

One of the problems his strategy brings is that it entails a heavy invasion of his private space. Mr Merton is never off duty. During the few hours a week when his wife has carers from a local voluntary organisation, he fits in his other jobs. Otherwise, Mr Merton is 'on-call' either in attending his wife or in dealing, together with her, with the many contacts and actions they are involved with. At times, it can become so claustrophobic that he has to retreat temporarily:

It is a 24-hour job, whatever happens, so if you get in a temper I normally go in the bedroom and I'll have a good bit of a scream. I come back out and say "forget" and then we sit down and forget about it and later we speak about it.

For the present, this lack of autonomous time may not matter. However, in the future, as his wife's care needs grow or his own condition may deteriorate, there might be a greater need to distinguish between the different aspects of his life, as a means of adapting to changing circumstances.

Family is best

This category of carers is characterised by a return from an outwardly oriented approach to caring to a more family-based care setting. This is often a defensive move because other strategies have become insufficient to meet the caring needs. It is often triggered by inadequacies of formal support, as experienced for example in the changeover from child to adult services.

The home-based strategy of carers in this group goes hand in hand with a willingness to participate in carer groups and disability associations. Unlike the West German cases, where caring is firmly located in the family context and external support remains marginal to the dynamics of caring, the reorientation towards family care does not result in isolation and retreat into the family sphere.

Mrs Buckley

East London borough

Mrs Buckley is the main carer for her 20-year-old adult daughter, Melanie, who lives at home and requires extensive assistance and supervision. Although Melanie has some sessions during the week at a day centre, she spends most of her time with her mother. The Buckleys have been active in the local carer organisation since Melanie's childhood. After many years of combining employment with Melanie's care, Mrs Buckley has to give up work because of her daughter's growing care needs and the lack of day-care cover. At present, Mrs Buckley finds it difficult to contemplate more independent living arrangements for her daughter.

Mrs Buckley comes from a strong Catholic working-class background, and is the youngest of a number of siblings. There are expectations in her family that she will remain at home and look after her ageing parents, a role traditionally allocated to the youngest daughter.

However, in a break with this tradition, Mrs Buckley leaves home in her late teens and starts a career in clothing retail, working her way up to the position of shop manager. She continues working even after she meets and marries Bob. The couple keep up their mobile, career-oriented lifestyle for a number of years.

Their only daughter, Melanie, is born when Mrs Buckley is in her thirties. Melanie has serious health problems which flare up at intervals, and severe learning disabilities. While the initial phase of diagnosis and treatment is a difficult period for the family, they eventually adjust and make use of available service provision. They have to fight for therapeutic treatment and services. For instance, just after Melanie is diagnosed, Mrs Buckley has to struggle for a referral to Great Ormond Street Hospital for Children:

> She [the doctor] said "We only send very sick children, really seriously sick children to Great Ormond Street" ... and so I said "I'll sit out in your waiting room and I'll wait until you do get in touch, I'm not going." So I sat there, Melanie's getting thirsty by that time.

Experiences like this remain a constant aspect in bringing up their daughter. Much of the family's energies in the following years are directed towards gaining the best possible services for their daughter. This is difficult in the late 1970s, as children's service provision in the East London borough is fragmented and of low quality. The Buckleys' strategy is to circumvent local services as much as possible. They find a lot of valuable support through their contacts with Great Ormond Street Hospital, where they are treated with much greater understanding and sympathy. Mrs Buckley manages to obtain a part-time job via such a contact, which allows her to work and look after Melanie at the same time.

The Buckleys also seek support among self-help and carer groups in the local area, participating actively in local disability, parents and carer support groups. This becomes an important part of their social life. They go regularly on a group holiday of families with disabled children, in a conscious attempt to break the isolation of families with disabilities.

During Melanie's teenage years, maintaining the balance between employment and care is more difficult to manage as Melanie's care needs and health problems become more complex. Mr Buckley used to share in the personal care of his daughter, but the couple both feel it is no longer appropriate for him to carry out this care, particularly after she starts menstruating. So Mrs Buckley becomes solely responsible for Melanie's personal care.

When Melanie transfers from children's services to adult services at the age of 18, her hours at the day centre are reduced, and Mrs Buckley can no longer fit her job around her daughter's day care. In a sudden decision, she gives up work:

> I was so upset about that [a friend's car accident], and I thought, "Oh, I'll pack up work" – I did it on the spur of the moment ... I did feel a bit, not bitter towards her [Melanie], but I just feel sometimes, "Oh, why did I have to pack up my job, because I liked it".

Mrs Buckley finds it increasingly difficult to extract herself from Melanie's care. Rather than having spare time for her self-help group and her various other social activities, she now finds herself coerced into the role of exclusive carer, drawing on family support – a role she has tried to avoid throughout her life.

Mrs Buckley experiences this as a traumatic dilemma. She is torn between the wish to relinquish some of the responsibilities of caring for her daughter, and her concern about the alternatives – respite and residential care:

> I want respite for her ... but I can't, I don't think anybody could look after her properly if she went into respite. And you get somebody who says, "Oh yes, we've got this one and we give out and we do this and do that" and they make it sound so easy for them, but they forget that I've worked in social services ... and they are not as efficient and as dedicated as they think they are.

Past experiences have coloured her view of formal service provision, making it even harder to make these difficult decisions about her daughter's future. The degree of her anxiety shows in that she becomes very upset and begins to cry at this point in the interview. Mrs Buckley knows that she ought to facilitate her daughter's independence. Emotionally, she clearly finds it hard to let her daughter go. She has not discussed her reservations with friends or other members of the self-help group. She cannot share them with her husband either. Mr Buckley is in favour of giving his daughter a more independent lifestyle in a residential unit. He is about to retire and would like to return to the more flexible lifestyle of their younger years. His plan for retirement is a world tour, something which Mrs Buckley is doubtful about: "Bob still thinks we are going and I really can't see how we can go ... and I would love, love, love to go".

The current situation causes tension between the couple. At this crucial juncture of her life as a carer, Mrs Buckley is rather unsupported.

Mrs Rushton

North London borough

Mrs Rushton cares for her husband, who has lived with multiple sclerosis (MS) for many years. Mr Rushton requires extensive assistance, most of which is provided by Mrs Rushton herself. Mrs Rushton spends much of her time maintaining her husband's daily routines, which enable him to maintain an independent and social life outside the confines of their flat. With the increasing dependency of her husband, this is becoming an oppressive and tiring regime for Mrs Rushton, at the cost of her own independence.

Mrs Rushton is in her early 60s. She is the sole carer of her husband, who has multiple sclerosis and now requires 24-hour care. The couple has three adult sons, who were brought up with their father's illness. Past resentments between father and sons mean that Mrs Rushton will not ask her children for even occasional assistance.

The Rushtons live on the ground floor of a purpose-built set of flats, which has some disability access. Mrs Rushton is assisted by two night nurses, who help her in getting her husband to bed each night. A nurse also comes once a week to give him a bath. The nursing assistance is necessary because of the complicated lifting procedure involved. Mr Rushton goes into respite care six weeks a year, paid for by the health authority. Occasionally he goes privately. Overall, most of the care is carried out by Mrs Rushton herself, according to a rigid routine:

> I have this routine and that daily routine is seven nights a week even when he doesn't go to the day centre.... Once he goes to the centre I can have my bath and I can get dressed you know, but my time is spent with him.

The couple's relationship is marked by tension and resentments about personal space and personal time. When arrangements for the interview are made, Mrs Rushton makes sure that her husband is at the day centre during the interview. When the end of the first interview coincides with her husband's return, she takes the interviewer to the station, smoking a cigarette on the way to expand the conversation for a little bit longer.

Mrs Rushton feels under constant pressure and undervalued in her efforts. She feels that her husband calls on her every few minutes to ask her to do things for him, such as move his legs, or give him drinks. Rather than addressing these simmering conflicts openly, they remain as a constant tension under the surface:

> I am constantly tired, and I can sit here and I'm longing and I just don't know how, I'm away, I'm asleep. But he'll wake me up to move his feet, so it doesn't matter, of a night-time or of an evening or even on a Sunday afternoon. If my eyes shut, it doesn't make any difference to him, he will still "Move my feet, push my feet!" – demanding. I appreciate on the other hand that he can't do these things himself, he has to have somebody do it, but I feel that, you know, "Think of me!".

Despite this, Mrs Rushton has rejected further services. She prefers to keep things as they are as the most effective way in 'getting through' the caring tasks. She experiences the nursing service as an intrusion into her private home sphere, as an invasion by strangers. At least by carrying out the personal care tasks herself, she can preserve her private space. Her evening routine is controlled by the visits of the night nurses, who will come at different times, making spontaneous change to the routine difficult:

> Your life is run without you having any say in it. You are beholden to them and also, you have people coming in a home.... I sometimes feel that I'm taken over, you know they come in ... but what I'm saying is my home is my own, I haven't got the privacy that I deserve. And then they say an Englishman's home is his castle, you've heard that expression?... Well it's shared, it's not my personal, private place ... they're coming in on my personal privacy.

The only regular breaks in this routine daily life come from her contacts with the MS groups the couple attend. In addition, Mrs Rushton insists on going to carer group meetings, because they are the few social contacts she still has. These regular social contacts are a lifeline for her:

> I do try to get to that because we end up having a moan and all our problems.... But we end up having a laugh as well, and I enjoy it, it is like a social.... Even at the day centre I meet up with other women there and

we end up having a laugh, we end up having more of a social and it gets you out of yourself.

However, the group is not the place to help her to seek a permanent solution to the daily pressures she feels. In this, she remains isolated within the private sphere, despite her outside contacts.

Mrs Rushton eventually suffers a breakdown, following a holiday.

It's a long journey by coach and I sat there, you're sat, and you're squashed up right, I think the emotion of the film [shown on the trip] I think I was a bit tearful and I sat there thinking how uncomfortable I was, and I thought this is how Rob is all the time and I came home depressed.

At present, there seems to be little chance of change or development in the situation, partly because Mrs Rushton is not prepared to allow further formal intervention in the home, either in the form of services or through wider social work support. Consequently, there is little planning of future care arrangements, a situation which may lead to crisis in time to come.

Reluctant transitions

The final category of carers is characterised by a process of renegotiating traditional strategies of family enclosure in favour of a more outwardly oriented strategy. Mrs Bally and Mrs Rajan move away from traditional family caring strategies by accepting formal services as a form of support. Mrs Rajan is assisted in this by a sympathetic social worker. Mrs Bally has no close contact with social work professionals; however, her own increasing frailty and age force her to seek alternatives to family care. For both carers this is a difficult process of personal transition.

In contrast to carers such as East German Herr Speyer or West German Frau Jakob, these British carers do not remain marooned in their situations, but are able to develop strategies which, over time, will bring about changes to make their situation more tolerable.

Mrs Rajan

> ### East London borough
>
> Mrs Rajan is in her 30s. She moves to Britain in her teens. Brought up in a traditional Indian family, she marries young and moves to East London to be near her husband's family. When her son is diagnosed as disabled, she struggles for a number of years to care for him and his small sister on her own. She is very isolated, with few contacts, no support services, and without assistance from her extended family. With the birth of her second son and through the contacts with school and nursery, she begins to make connections in the local community and becomes more outgoing. She seeks help from social services and begins work as a nursery assistant.

Mrs Rajan spends her childhood in Kenya, leading a secluded life. The family moves to Britain when she is in her early teens. Her marriage to a bus driver at the age of 17 separates her from her own family. She moves to East London borough, expecting to become part of his extended family.

However, the relationship with her in-laws does not develop well. She becomes isolated and lonely. Her isolation is confounded when she has two children in quick succession. The little boy, Bavesh, is disabled from birth and develops behaviour problems in childhood. This increases her isolation, and for a number of years Mrs Rajan leads a completely isolated existence in her flat, with little other contact than with her husband and her children:

> I used to keep them in the cot and quickly go in the shop, you know. Quick with milk and come back, you know. But I feel really bad, feel guilty. If anything happens to them I get the blame, yeah. My husband found out that I had been doing this and we had a good argument, you know. He said "You'd better stop it".

When her husband realises the extent of her isolation, he begins to participate in the care of their children. He takes greater responsibility in the home, and participates in the housework chores. The marriage is becoming more of a partnership.

Mrs Rajan finds adjustments and change difficult. She has few outside contacts and copes with her difficult situation on her own. Her isolation is exacerbated by the continued difficulties she has with her husband's family, who exclude her and offer little help. Her main contact is with her own family, who can only visit at intervals. She feels she is marginalised in her own community, not the least because of Bavesh's difficult behaviour in public:

> See even if there is a wedding invitation either I go or he [her husband] goes.... You can't take him [Bavesh] there because he never sits down. He's always singing and sometimes he is in a bad mood, he might start swearing you know ... it's really tough sometimes, you feel all depressed at times, but there is nothing you can do.

The slow process of change in Mrs Rajan's caring strategy is triggered through the birth of their third child, a boy, in 1990. The couple have discussed the risks of a further pregnancy, but Mrs Rajan insists on attempting to have another child. Although this change occurs over many years, it is as if the second son gives her the freedom to explore new tangents in her life. An important landmark in this transformation is confrontation with her in-laws in general, and her mother-in-law in particular.

When her second son starts school, the head teacher of the school invites her to become a nursery assistant in the reception class. Mrs Rajan is delighted with this role and is now considering taking up training for a career in this field. The increased contact with the school also brings the opportunity for greater contact with social services. The Rajans build up a good relationship with Mrs Rajan's social worker, who is Indian herself. She becomes a source of advice, discussing future care options for Bavesh. He is now aged 12, and the family contemplates permanent residential care.

Mrs Rajan expected to fit into a traditional British-Indian lifestyle, particularly in living with the help and support provided through the extended family context. However, the circumstances of her family life in effect pull her into the nuclear family unit, with much more individualised patterns of role division and obligation. The care needs of her older son isolate her further as a mother and carer. It is only when she can finally fulfil her own expectations as the mother of a healthy boy that she comes to terms with the changed circumstances and can move on.

Mrs Bally

North London borough

Together with her now retired husband, Mrs Bally is the main carer for her son Peter (29), the youngest of her three children. He has moderate learning problems and physical disabilities. During the 1980s, in Peter's teenage years, Mrs Bally also cares for her mother. Because of her caring commitment to her son, Mrs Bally reluctantly agrees for her mother to go into residential accommodation. At the time of the interviews in 1995, Peter lives at home. Mrs Bally is now reluctantly looking into residential care for her son, because of her own age and health problems.

Mrs Bally's childhood is characterised by a disrupted family life, which involves a spell in an orphanage when she is still young. She decides early on that she wants some qualifications: " ... I realised I really wanted to do something a bit better with my life and I started nursing".

Mrs Bally starts nursing training in the later part of the Second World War as a recruit to the war effort. She qualifies as a paediatric nurse. She marries in the 1950s and has four children, all boys. She fits her job around the family by working in geriatric wards or residential homes for the elderly. Peter, the fourth child, is born when Mrs Bally is 42. Mrs Bally notices that something is wrong immediately:

> When I asked, nobody would tell me immediately. They said "you'll see a paediatrician before you leave the hospital". However, by the time I saw the paediatrician I'd already told my husband and my sons what was wrong with him.

When they receive the diagnosis of disability, Mrs Bally makes immediate plans for how to deal with the situation:

> And I said to my husband ... go home and tell all our friends and neighbours what is wrong with the baby. You know, they could come and see us and I didn't want people shocked or anything, you know, to sort of look at the pram and go away thinking there was something wrong. I wanted them to know and accept him for what he was.

In the early years, Peter's development is encouraging and the family increase their efforts to enable their son to achieve through good schooling and training.

> The excitement when he was little was when he did something himself, you know, when he first walked – that was great excitement. I remember, my older son had been to choir practice; he came home and we said: "We've got something to show you". We said to Peter: "Go to Brian". And I can see it in my mind now, he was so excited, he leapt up in the air, you know – thought it was wonderful to see him walk, because we worked very hard with him when he was born in encouraging him in everything.

When Mrs Bally cannot find a place in an integrated nursery in her borough, she finds a place for Peter in the neighbouring one, to ensure that he can participate in early learning. The Ballys are drawn into the activities of the nursery, organising fundraising and starting carers' meetings. They try out different integrative schooling schemes. But this proves to be too difficult and Peter attends a special school. The family become activists, campaigning for better local services via local health groups and carers groups. The Ballys participate in the emerging self-help and community groups which spring up in the late 1960s, and they benefit from improving facilities and changing attitudes towards disabled children.

Mrs Bally returns to work, in the belief that Peter now receives the 'specialist' attention he requires through formal channels. She fits her job around the children's school times:

> I always thought, I will be at home when my children come home from school or anything because I felt if they had anything to tell you, they'd tell you directly they came in the door. If you weren't there they wouldn't tell you – it's gone and it could be very important.

While the parents are actively organising better services for Peter, there is a tendency to overprotect him within the family. He never learns personal care tasks – even today his father brushes his teeth. Peter's response to this cocoon of family protection is to develop a habit of 'wandering', that is leaving the house and not returning. He is always found, but the habit creates a worry for his parents.

Problems begin to arise after Peter finishes compulsory schooling and spends increasing time at home. At the age of 16, he can only go to a day centre part-time. The family find funding for other activities difficult, either because of the cost or because of the regulations attached to further services:

> We got a young woman, didn't we, and she used to come and take him out once a week even and they said, eh, we would pay and they would send us the money once a month [amusement]. After we spent a hundred pounds, they wrote and said it was not for that, it was for somebody doing something for him at home. Well, you know, that wasn't what we wanted – we can do things with him indoors.

Peter becomes increasingly dependent on his parents because the adult disability services and entitlements are much more limited, and choices are more restricted. While the Ballys continue to pursue benefits and additional financial assistance whenever possible, Peter's life begins to be more confined to his home environment. When Mrs Bally's mother becomes ill and develops dementia during this transition period, Mrs Bally cannot take on the extensive caring role she would want to. In the end, she has to admit her mother to a psychiatric long-stay hospital:

> Then finally they phoned me and said, you know, there is a permanent place for your mother ... I mean it was a relief really and she was well looked after.

For the first time, Mrs Bally begins to see herself as a carer. Before this episode, "we didn't consider ourselves as carers, you know. He was ours." The Ballys begin to claim greater financial support for their son and investigate alternative services for him. After Mr Bally retires, he takes over the personal care. While the couple find it difficult to contemplate change, they also know that ultimately the current situation cannot continue. They start discussing alternative arrangements. It is an emotionally painful process, but Mrs Bally recognises the limitations of her ability to carry on:

> I suppose as I got older really and when you're younger you don't consider these things because you're fit and well, and I suppose when you get older you suddenly realise that it's more a burden to you what you're doing.

The couple are now in regular contact with social workers and the social services department about Peter's future, and are edging towards the possibility of letting Peter enter into more independent living. It is not an easy process for either of the parents:

> We know it's got to come at some time, but it's very, very hard to make the decision. We don't want to do it yet, but we know that's got to come at some time, in the not too distant future. You can't plan your life, you can't plan when you're gonna die, I suppose this is the – the hardest [she cries].

Comparisons

The British cases are characterised by highly individualised carer strategies which highlight different points of a continuum of informal care rather than representing mutually exclusive categories. Unlike the German cases, British carers transcend the boundaries between public, private and social spheres, enabling them to change and adapt their strategies according to changing circumstances, with the help of social networks and formal support services at different points in their caring careers.

At one end of the spectrum, carers like Mr Allahm and Mr Merton develop their new social identities through their disability work and church involvement. Mr Allahm mobilises his experience of and commitment to his church community to create a support network for his own private caring situation. Mr Merton's caring role and disability work allow him to bring aspects of his previous life and personality into the foreground, aspects which hitherto have been only tangential to his life.

At the other end of the spectrum, Mrs Buckley and Mrs Rushton have withdrawn into the roles of 'traditional' informal carers. Both women still have outside contacts and retain links with self-help and carer groups. Of the two cases, Mrs Buckley's 'withdrawal' appears more dramatic, in that she moves from a strategy of outside involvement and activism, giving up her job and active involvement with her community groups, to become the exclusive carer to her daughter. Although Mrs Rushton is not politically active, she has maintained her links with support groups throughout her longstanding caring career, for a much needed break. Both women are not as isolated in their current situation as some of the West German carers, and they retain social contact and support.

Mrs Bally and Mrs Rajan's cases are located between these extremes. For these carers, accepting formal services in the form of residential care and social work support is part of a slow process of moving away from family-based care and into increasing cooperation with formal service provision. For both women it implies a cultural departure from private, family-based caring towards greater outward orientation. While this is a new development for Mrs Rajan, for Mrs Bally it means connecting with the childhood period in the care of her son, when the family adopted a more outgoing approach to care. In the longer term, it allows their children greater independence and the prospect of independent development. It also brings a degree of freedom, which they have not experienced over a long period of time.

In comparison with the West German cases, British carers show a greater degree of flexibility and adaptability in caring arrangements, which takes them beyond narrow, normative definitions of care. None of the carers presented in the British case studies are 'wedded' to their adopted caring strategies. Over time, all the carers have undergone processes of change and have adapted their strategies not only according to circumstances, but also according to the changing needs of the cared-for person. Mrs Buckley responds to Melanie's changing needs during her adolescence by adopting the role of full-time carer. While Mrs Buckley regrets the loss of her own freedom in this process, taking on caring for her daughter brings some continuity and security to her daughter's daily life. Also, it does not preclude the possibility that, in time, Mrs Buckley will be able to accept further changes in the caring context and that Melanie will move away from home and live independently.

In contrast to the East German cases, in which carers have found themselves propelled into participating in outward orientation, British carers retain greater control over their own caring pathways. Mrs Rajan has space to develop her relationship with formal services at her own pace and in her own time. Objectively, she clearly needed support from early on, but may have found it difficult to tolerate direct intervention in her private family world at an earlier time. Her contact with the 'public world of social care services' comes at a personally 'appropriate' time, when her self-esteem has recovered and has enabled her to embark on this development. The intervention of her Asian social worker is crucial in facilitating the process.

The cost of this flexibility and self-determination lies in the fragility of the British caring arrangements over time. While in the East and West German cases, carers tend to be pulled into one particular caring pattern, the British carers find that they have to adapt their caring solutions frequently. Mrs Buckley takes on the role of informal carer only reluctantly after Melanie has to leave child health services. In these new circumstances, the networks of support that Mrs Buckley has cultivated over the years, and the services she has fought for, are not enough to sustain the comparative independence of her own lifestyle as a working mother and carer. Mr Allahm and Mr Merton also find it difficult to hold a balance between the competing demands of the public and private spheres. Mr Allahm is actively seeking to recruit his sister-in-law as his permanent house companion and carer for his wife. The carefully developed caring strategies seem to be less stable than in some of the German cases.

Service intervention and informal care

In Britain, more so than for their East and West German counterparts, the experience of carers has been moulded by continued changes in service provision and structure. Despite or perhaps as a result of the frequency of change, carers have found that choices of formal service have remained limited, largely fragmented and unresponsive to their individual needs. Mrs Rushton has to accommodate her daily routines around nurses' visits. Mrs Bally finds that the services offered to her son do not bring any relief for her, but require further organisation and effort on her part.

While these experiences echo the complaints of West German carers about unresponsive and bureaucratic services, British carers also have to remain 'available' to bridge shortfalls in services and to fight constantly for service improvements. Indeed, many of the 'victories' in terms of improved services have been the result of persistent fights for improvements, at least from the perspective of carers themselves. Formal services remain residual and difficult to access. Consequently, carers are left with the subjective perception that the ultimate safeguard for adequate care remains with families and the informal carer.

So far, post-1990 community care seems to have done little to change either the perception or the reality of informal care. Carers do not report greater support as the result of assessments or through improved service provision. Rather, worries about cuts and financial assessments of eligibility are common. The Mertons, for example, have to undergo frequent assessments to determine his continued eligibility for items of equipment for adaptations to their home.

In both boroughs, there have been cuts to services and provision has been streamlined. Mr Rushton's respite care, a lifeline for Mrs Rushton, is strictly rationed to a number of visits a year, and may be further reduced as a result of a shortage of respite beds in the area. Day-care facilities for

Melanie Buckley and Peter Bally also remain inadequate, reducing their chances of personal development and meaningful social activity.

Perversely, the way out in all three cases would be residential care. As adults, Melanie Buckley and Peter Bally are eligible to move into some form of residential accommodation. Similarly, Mr Rushton may already qualify for a residential care place, given his deteriorating health (although it may be difficult to find a suitable place for him in the short term). Clearly, this is not an acceptable option for the families at present. In these situations, there is no 'middle way', in which formal care services can be truly supportive of the particular needs and requirements of intensifying individual caring needs.

Exceptionally to the above cases, community care *has* contributed much to a change in Mrs Rajan's situation. As increased support for minority ethnic carers is one of the priority areas in East London borough's community care strategy, Mrs Rajan has benefited greatly from the work with her Asian social worker. She has been able to call on her frequently, and receives the long-term attention she requires to help her through the personally difficult period of transition. Clearly, the multicultural approach of East London borough and the resources brought into this strategy have helped to bring carers such as Mrs Rajan into the mainstream of community care.

A further barrier in making the new policies acceptable lies in the deeply seated mistrust of the quality of care that can be provided through formal services. All carers' accounts contain experiences of inadequate standards of care and the callousness of professionals, which have eroded trust in the system and make it difficult for carers to change their perceptions about public provision as a source of valid care.

Mrs Bally and Mrs Buckley are wary of the prospect of permanent residential care for their children. As a nurse on a geriatric ward, Mrs Bally has first-hand experience of the 'old system' of residential care during the 1960s and 1970s. This has coloured her perception of residential care. Although she finally accepted residential care for her mother, for Mrs Bally the legacy of her own experiences makes it even harder to contemplate alternative care arrangements for her son. Her perceptions of the shortcomings of residential care may be unfairly prejudiced, but they influence her perspective of choices in an important way. In contrast, Mrs Rajan is expecting that her son will live in residential care in the future. Unlike other carers, her 'history' with formal service providers is relatively short and largely supportive. It is not surprising that she should be much more open to the formal care services.

Community care operates within the continuum of a catalogue of reforms and changes to the system, which many of the carers have personal experiences of, and which form the background to the continued perceptions and prejudices about state service provision. And unlike the situation in East Germany, where the failings of formal service provision were much more crass, the British welfare system does not have the dimension of closure, which might allow carers to view new service structures less suspiciously.

The role of social contacts and networks

For the carers in the British study, participation in social support groups provides spaces for community action, social support and personal development. Mrs Buckley and Mrs Bally are active in their local areas, working on several campaigns and in a series of groups. Mrs Rajan develops social links through her contacts with the school and the local area.

Mr Merton's and Mr Allahm's 'interpretation' of caring as work and as a community activity has transformed the private caring activity into a 'public' occupation; this distinguishes their approach from the traditional female sphere of caring. Mr Allahm, for example, involves himself so much in his church that he is now looking for a 'replacement' carer to look after his wife, so he can "get on with some work". For Mr Merton, the contact in the community and his political campaigning with his wife reinforce the equality between the couple and provide additional common ground in their relationship.

As with the West German cases, participating in these social spheres also has limitations: for most carers in the British study, the social networks and contacts with carer and disability groups do not relieve personal dilemmas in care. Being part of her local campaigning group does not solve the fundamental problems Mrs Bally experiences in reaching a more permanent solution for her son's care. It remains a private problem. Social support networks do not seem to provide a framework within which these problems can be successfully addressed.

Mrs Buckley, although active in her local carer group, does not use the social contacts and networks for developing Melanie's independence. In recent years, the family has withdrawn much more into the private family sphere, and links with former group members are purely private. Like Mr Allahm, she is also restricted by the sheer time commitment that continued involvement would require – as her daughter's care needs increase, she simply does not have the time and flexibility to continue her work in the group. Mrs Rushton comments on the limitations of the social sphere of carers networks: "I only go there for the company. It gets me out of the house".

It is clearly not easy to combine informal care and active social embeddedness successfully over time. As the Hegemann family in West Germany shows, there is a real danger of support group 'fatigue', which can result in withdrawal from the social support sphere. It is not clear how active Mrs Bally, Mrs Buckley or Mrs Rushton were in their respective campaign and support groups in the past. From a contemporary perspective, their participation appears more passive and casual, and not a potential catalyst for personal development or change. This suggests that support groups and campaign groups have a limited capacity for engendering and facilitating personal change on a large scale.

Conclusion

The culture of care in Britain moves within a triad of private, public and social dimensions, in which caring is located within individualised strategies. Family strategies and histories feature strongly in determining the adaptation processes. The social sphere of self-help and carers organisations and networks is also widely developed, allowing carers (under some relatively transient conditions) to participate and be active in their social and political communities.

British carers are positioned between the internal pull of the West German and the external push of the East German culture of care. Unlike the West German carers, British carers are able to transcend the dichotomy of formal and informal care, and the choices they make about care do not seem to cause such extensive personal conflicts as they do among some of the West German carers.

British carers seem less committed to existing social welfare institutions. Instead, they use the norms of their own life histories and personal experiences to carve out their caring strategies. In contrast to the more traditional West German cases, this individualised pattern of care places a particular onus on the ability of personal and private resources to create an individual path through the caring experience, enriching and transforming the life experiences of carers in the process.

Potentially, this close involvement with the social sphere also offers British carers the chance to embrace values of a lively and viable social sphere of mutual support, self-fulfilment and transformative action (Williams, 1993). However, there are limitations to such a process. The continuing changes and instability of the formal welfare system mean that carers are thrown back to the private sphere of care in order to compensate for the shortfalls of the system. As a consequence, there is little space to work towards longer-term goals of change in the informal sphere. Carers such as Mrs Buckley and Mrs Bally demonstrate that, if the necessity arises, carers can and will easily retreat into the private sphere if circumstances require them to. It is therefore not surprising that the wide network of voluntary and self-help groups functions only to provide limited social support and contact for carers.

Above all, the British cases illustrate the need for a balance among private, social and public dimensions in informal care. Britain has a strong tradition of informal care, underpinned by extensive academic and policy reports which testify to the robustness and commitment of informal carers to their roles and tasks. It also has a diverse and active self-help movement, which can provide the necessary social support for carers. However, as long as formal services do not provide the back-up to informal care to develop sustainable care strategies, the chance for permanent change and development remains remote.

Note

[1] Community care affects a growing number of people. In 1996, a million households in Britain received some form of home care, while 150,000 people aged over 65 lived in residential care (Department of Health, 1996). Financially, the number of people contributing to their own care costs has increased substantially, by 450,000 between 1984 and 1994 (Joseph Rowntree Foundation, 1996). This increasing financial burden is felt most severely within residential care provision, in which full charges apply for savings over £10,000 and property values over £16,000. The Royal Commission which investigated the issues of long-term care provision and finance reported late in 1999, and recommended a further overhaul of the financing principle of care, including higher thresholds (Royal Commission on Long-term Care, 1999). At the time of writing, the government's response is still awaited, but is not expected to overhaul the funding structure fundamentally. It is unlikely to address issues of funding community-based services.

FIVE

Biography and caring

Introduction

As we have seen, carers respond very differently to the challenges and demands of caring. Structural factors and external contingencies influence the way caring is experienced and responded to, but the personal dimension has an equally important impact on the way informal care develops over time. It is this dimension that we explore here, drawing out the personal meanings of caring and highlighting their relationship with social dimensions of welfare. We return to the different case studies, considering cases across the three societies and expanding the themes raised in the previous chapters.

The literature of caregiving has not as yet produced a 'holistic' model of caring which could satisfactorily theorise its dynamic and multidimensional nature (Nolan et al, 1996, p 2). Rather, research has centred on specific dimensions, such as carers' experiences, coping, and the emotional and physical consequences of caring (Lewis and Meredith, 1988; Opie, 1994; Twigg and Atkin, 1994; Nolan and Grant, 1993; Willoughby and Keating, 1991).

Issues of process and change in caring relationships have tended to be centred on stages of transition, while temporal and longitudinal aspects remain under-theorised (see for example Wilson, 1989; Nolan et al, 1996). An exception to this is the work by Keady and Nolan (1994); they explored the biographical dimension of caring and identified six distinct phases in the care of long-term dementia patients from a nursing perspective.

Our own approach emphasises the biographical dimension, relating caring to a longitudinal life-course perspective. In this approach, care is a biographical project, in which past life events and experiences, expectations and aspirations for the future, as well as the present circumstances, are formatively involved in the development of informal care. As the case studies presented in the previous three chapters indicate, caring and being a carer is actively negotiated and constantly renegotiated, and carers are active participants in creating their own situations and circumstances.

Three ideas inform our understanding and subsequent analysis of the biographical accounts of carers: biography, trajectory and strategy. Through these concepts we explore caring as a process that is structured both by internal dynamics and by external circumstances. The chapter begins by introducing the main theoretical concepts underpinning the approach used. In the second and third sections, the case studies are re-examined in the light of these concepts, particularly in relation to how caring trajectories are translated into active caring strategies. In the last section, we discuss the implications of our approach for service intervention.

Concepts

The starting point of a biographical analysis of care is the premise that caring is a significant life-course event, regardless of the length of the caring activity or its eventual outcome. As such, carers need to place caring experiences and activities within a context of wider life experiences. Over the life course of an individual, significant life events are ordered along a continuum of past, present and future perspectives. Through this, meaning can be assigned to these events without damaging the continuity of a biographical understanding of the self (Rosenthal, 1993). Caring is part of a flow of biographical development which is connected to a person's past and has relevance to the future. While the project of caring and being a carer is not in itself pre-planned or programmed, the experiences and actions flowing from it are biographically shaped. Caring is enmeshed in a web of personal and social relationships which form the social fabric of a person's life.

Our understanding of caring is somewhat different to concepts of care and care work that are based on the contingency of the care needs and care services (see for example, Twigg and Atkin, 1994). In our understanding, caring is an active and potentially transformative process, in which carers need to adjust their perspectives of their own lives to accommodate caring into their own life experiences. The decision to care may arise as a contingency; however, as it develops it becomes an active process, which requires a personal response and biographical work. Caring in the informal sphere is therefore actively 'created', rather than passively 'endured'. At the same time, the experience of care is fuelled by the dynamics of everyday practice and is not necessarily self-reflective. The 'creative' dimension is most clearly demonstrated by carers such as Frau Luchtig, Mr Merton or Frau Hamann, who have taken on the carer role as a 'biographical project'. For these carers, caring is self-consciously linked to their sense of self and identity. While others may not reflect on this dimension explicitly, as for example Frau Alexander and Frau Meissner, the experience nevertheless has meaning beyond their day-to-day caring routine.

Theoretically, this perspective on care links with the notion of 'biographical work' developed by Fischer-Rosenthal (2000). As society is increasingly losing the normative constraints of social values and obligations of the past, one's own biography and life experiences are becoming increasingly significant in mapping one's life courses. He argues that this process implies continued 'biographical work' as the basis for informed and strategic agency. The continued re-examination of the past in the light of new experiences and events allows the individual to develop strategies for dealing with the current and future social world. Biography and biographical work become a resource for structuring everyday life. 'Reworking' one's biography in the light of caring is part of a larger process of continuous biographical work throughout the life course. The notion of 'biographical work' as an active process resembles the notion of 'emotion work' developed by Hochschild (1979), who argues that there is an active relationship between self and the social world, centred on the active management of feeling states in everyday interactions.

The second notion used in this chapter is that of trajectory. The idea of a trajectory has been developed by the sociologists Corbin and Strauss (1988) to describe the consequences of long-term and chronic illness on subjectivity and self. Riemann and Schütze (1991) develop the term to explore the impact of a person's illness on life-course expectations and identity (p 339). They argue that as individuals we are enmeshed in a web of social relations, which form the background to generalised life-course trends and along which life events can be ordered. The idea of trajectory is that this can be disrupted by a chain of events which is outside the control of the individual and characterised by "a disorder of expectation, orientation, and relationship to world and identity" (p 340). Trajectory refers to the process of biographically 'losing control' over one's life, even if only temporarily, and with it the ordered sequence of existing identity and personal and social relationships. Pulling back from this threatened state of personal anomie requires a process of active adaptation to the trajectory, and with it intense biographical work.

As the counter-concept to trajectory, we are using the idea of 'strategy' as the process by which the disruptions to biographical mould caused by the caring trajectories are healed and the impact of the life-changing events is at least contained (Bury, 1982). It is about gaining control over the events and integrating them into the carers' own life paths, opening up new future perspectives for life within and beyond caring.

'Strategy' refers to the purposeful way in which people manoeuvre towards a particular goal through a set of complicated circumstances, sometimes over an extended period. Originally developed as a concept for understanding wars (von Clausewitz, 1968), the notion of strategy has found applications in, for example, game theory. Used as a way of understanding the behaviour of actors for achieving a strategic outcome, strategy implies the use of a whole variety of 'choices' about how to 'implement' the strategy and how to adapt to the ever-changing and 'turbulent field' of social action (Emery, 1969). In this definition, the emphasis is clearly on the rational manipulation of behaviour, for a predetermined purpose, sometimes over the longer term.

The term conveys a sense of control and purposefulness and a notion of reflectivity and self-knowledge. Used in this context, caring strategy acknowledges the active part played by carers in developing caring over time. The strategy employed by carers such as Frau Hager (whose case is described in a cameo at the beginning of the book) is to maintain her and her mother's independence and emotional well-being in the face of her own deteriorating health and her mother's frailty. She is very proactive in retaining her contacts with friends, acquaintances and former work colleagues by inviting them to her home and by arranging regular meetings. She supervises rather than carries out her mother's care, and is determined to retain her own flat. This can be seen as a deliberate strategy to counteract the danger of isolation and dependency in her situation as a carer and unemployed disabled person in the post-unification era. Through this strategy, Frau Hager retains control of her situation, her lifeworld.

Many of the day-to-day decisions taken by carers are not deliberate strategic choices or self-reflective decisions. Nevertheless, they become understandable within overall patterns of responding to life events, established over the life course. Mrs Buckley's decision to quit her job, for example, is a spontaneous reaction rather than a rationally considered choice. It is consistent with her pattern of returning to a situation of family enclosure as an alternative to the previous, more outwardly oriented care strategy. Similarly, Frau Jakob's rejection of residential care for her husband is understandable as part of her commitment to family-based care. In this context, the term relates more to that used in psychotherapy, which refers to 'unconscious strategies' uncovered through the psychotherapeutic process. There, it refers to practices and patterns which structure everyday life and decisions, but which are not fully self-consciously understood or always coherently applied (Haley, 1963). It is through the therapeutic process that these strategies are made conscious and their place in the life pattern made explicit.

Biographical strategies refer to the process of biographical adaptation, of finding a new identity as a carer, of linking one's new role to one's former life, both as a deliberate and self-reflective course of action and as a means of everyday practice, embedded in the biographical patterns of past experiences. Biographical strategy influences the way that carers negotiate the caring process within the constraints and opportunities of family relations, service provision and financial contexts – in short, how they find a way of adapting to caring within the circumstances in which they find themselves. We identify three categories of biographical strategies: those carers who integrate caring into their previous life courses and continue their biographical paths; carers for whom caring engenders a new biographical direction; and a third category of carers who combine elements of continuity and change. We have named these basic patterns of adaptation 'biographical continuity', 'biographical change' and 'parallel lives'.

An important aspect of the success of carers' strategies over time is the degree of insight they develop over their situation, how consciously carers perceive caring not simply as an activity, but also as a 'biographical' event. This reflexivity, "the subjects' explicit understanding of themselves and their situations", has an impact on the longer-term outcome of the success of the caring strategies (Chamberlayne and Rustin, 1999, p 21).

We established the connection between the different biographical spheres, trajectory and strategy through the use of the biographical case study method. The introductory prompt at the beginning of the interviews (see Chapter One, Introduction) only invites carers to reflect on caring as a life event, without insisting on such an account. The response to the prompt was varied. A few carers cast their whole life within the context of their current lives as carers. Other interviewees did not make the connection between their current caring activities and their past lives, and talked about either their lives or their situation as carers. The method of case reconstruction circumvents these limitations in biographical self-accounting by reconstructing the lived as well as the narrated life stories (Rosenthal, 1993). It is a process of double reconstruction, in which interviewees reconstruct their life in the interview, and the researcher reconstructs the life story on the two levels of lived and told life (Chamberlayne and King, 1996).

Clearly, the case history we have developed from each case is a highly interpreted version of a person's actual life, and should be read as a 'case' rather than as representing the complete richness of a person's life. Our analytical work is bounded by the limited information available within a context of time-limited interview, and can also only detect hints of emotional motivations underlying the life experiences (for a broader discussion of analysis of subjectivity in social theory see Domingues, 2000). However, the material obtained through the method is rich enough to reconstruct aspects of the life course and write it into a 'case study', much more than semi-structured interviewing could achieve. Through the comparison with other cases, we can extract the overarching themes of carers' strategies. Our presentation of the case material is our way of bringing the cases to life.

In the next section of this chapter, we discuss the case studies in terms of the biographical meaning that caring poses, exploring the different motivational patterns that inform 'choosing' a biographical response.

The last section of the chapter discusses the opportunities and limitations these orientations have as adaptation strategies, and their effects on the ability of the carer to engage with the outside world and on adaptability to facing change in the caring context. Finally, we discuss lessons for policy makers and social policy intervention.

Carer trajectories

Caring as biographical continuity

> Yes, yes I always say, I was born for it, I was the oldest and the responsibility was put into my cradle for everything that happened. It stayed like this, my siblings, I always had to do a lot for my brothers and my parents, they always pushed me into everything [one-second pause].

Frau Luchtig's opening remarks in her interview acknowledge the lifelong significance her caring has for her. Before anything else has been said about her current circumstances, her current life and her caring activity, she highlights it as a continuous and determining feature in her life. It is something which has meaning well beyond her current role as the carer of her frail elderly mother. She cared for her siblings and took care of the business interests of her parents. Her role as carer to her frail mother is an extension of her role as the dutiful daughter, a role she has fulfilled throughout her life. It is, as argued in Chapter Two, a role that she resents bitterly and is at the root of her conflict with her mother.

It is the formative theme in her life, her life's mould, particularly from a contemporary perspective. Currently, as the carer of her frail mother, this 'carer' role poses a threat to her musical and artistic activities in the local orchestra and as a sculptor. To Frau Luchtig, being a carer is the continuous pursuit of other people's interest and well-being at the cost of her own interests, aspirations and happiness.

For Frau Jakob, too, being a carer has life-course significance: to her it has become a standard of family obligation and loyalty. Taking on the caring responsibility during the last five years of her husband's life has been a lonely activity, largely unsupported. However, to her it means the continuation of her life theme and personal value system in which "families look out for each other": it is what she would have done for her parents, and corresponds to her understanding of family obligation. She continues living to this standard, regardless of the advice she received from health professionals and irrespective of the fact that her family – her sisters, son and brother-in-law – do not provide support. Unlike Frau Luchtig who regrets her 'lost' life, Frau Jakob upholds her complete commitment to caring, even after the death of her husband.

For both women, the experience of being a carer is emotionally fraught and negative. Nevertheless, within the caring trajectory, the strategies also provide a comprehensive narrative to the self and the outside world. Within her narrative, Frau Luchtig can contain the emotional antagonism towards her mother and maintain her role of victim of her parents. Frau Jakob also has the means of tolerating her increasingly isolated existence, because it allows her to live out her ideology of traditional family loyalty. Both women represent a group of (female) carers, who continue their lifelong biographical path, characterised by family care and lifelong caring activities. While they bring very different motivations and experiences to caring, Frau Luchtig and Frau Jakob have extended their traditional roles to accommodate the illness and disability of kin.

Another subgroup among these carers is parents who care for children with disability. Carers such as Mrs Bally describe their caring as continuing childcare roles. They are motivated by preserving a 'normal' family life. Providing a close and intimate family environment is born out of Mrs Bally's wish not to repeat her own disruptive childhood. Caring maintains her strong family life and integrates the care her son Peter requires within the wider family context. Similarly, Frau Schumann (another carer from

West Germany) decides to keep her son at home despite his disruptive behaviour which puts her other children at considerable risk. In answering the question of why they do not opt for residential care, she replies:

> If we put him there, we could not have visited in the next few months. We would not be allowed to buy him clothes. Only on his birthday would we be allowed to give him a present. We could only visit him once a month and in the holidays he would be allowed to visit for a week, and my husband and I said, "... no, then he is gone completely and we won't see him at all".

Both women strongly identify with their family roles, although the caring arrangement is threatening the family unit at different points. This affirmative power in a carer identity, linking up different stages of life, is also clearly demonstrated by two of the male carers, Herr Speyer from East Germany and Mr Allahm from Britain. For both men, caring offers them continuity in managing their family affairs. As Mr Speyer has managed his wife's epilepsy throughout their marriage, her dependency insulates him from the social changes to family life and gender roles in the emerging East German society. For Mr Allahm, the carer role is also a confirmation of the continuity in their relationship in an otherwise significantly disrupted life; being a carer provides renewed permanence against the unsettled lifestyle which has characterised their married life. Caring as a man also gives them a foothold and esteem in their social settings and milieus, generating support, respect and sympathy – something which some of the female carers may not receive to the same degree.

Carers who manage to continue caring as part of their overall biographical mould invest a significant portion of their selves and their identity into caring. This can be a powerful resource in maintaining care, often over a very long period. Frau Jakob and Herr Speyer manage to keep their spouses at home in the most adverse and difficult circumstances with minimal support. Through their determination to see their roles through to the very end, they actually provide the equivalent of 24-hour intensive nursing care.

Change and the life-course perspective

The second group of carers has taken a different path in adapting to the challenge of caring as a biographical project. Their personal lives have undergone a significant shift through the caring process itself. Sometimes this shift is sudden, rupturing aspects of the person's self, resulting in a change in their biographical outlook. Sometimes the process is much more gradual. In either case, they result in a shift in the biography through personal development and orientation.

A most dramatic process of personal adaptation is that of Mr Merton, the disability campaigner from East London. Mr Merton used to drift from job to job, without real roots in his East London community. His own disability and that of his wife have politicised his outlook and opened new dimensions in his biographical horizons.

Frau Meissner and Frau Hildebrand (from East Germany) have become active disability rights campaigners, using their expertise in fighting the authorities to help other people, and changing their own lives in the process. Frau Meissner vividly describes the Herculean effort in her many years of campaigning, though she tells her story in self-effacing terms. Between the towering opposed forces of good and evil, she has learned to act against the overwhelming odds of the East German system to achieve her daughter's integration. In the process she has become a highly competent, enterprising and well-informed person, an informal carer who has become a professional disability campaigner. She has given a profile to the 'invisible mother' of East German society, and in the process carved out a public, autonomous identity.

Frau Meissner's path turned her into an outgoing and adventurous member of her own circle of able-bodied and disabled friends. Frau Hildebrand even develops her campaign work into professional activity. She is now employed by the disability lobbying group she co-founded after draining years as an isolated carer with a growing family. Similarly to Frau Meissner, she has had to fight the East German authorities for appropriate services for her autistic daughter and has had to endure widespread ignorance and prejudice in attitudes among professionals. Through the shared experiences and collective of disability self-help, her family has not only found acceptance, support and information, but Frau Hildebrand has also developed a new understanding of her daughter's condition:

> There was a big meeting here in Leipzig, organised by the Disability Association and there was a learning disability group. For many parents it is a positive thing, that their child is autistic, because it is something special, not quite the mundane mental disability. If you are precise, it is a mental disability just like any other. If you struggle to take that idea on board, you can view disability with different eyes.

Not everybody develops a public persona. Frau Planck's, Frau Alexander's and Mrs Rajan's process of biographical reorientation has centred on personal development and changes in their personal lives. Frau Planck is a young, single mother with three children (her case is presented as a cameo at the beginning of the book). Frau Planck's relationships with the fathers of her children have not worked out, and the children are only in irregular contact with them. Her own childhood was difficult and she ran away from home on several occasions. Today, she has no contact with her own family and so is very much on her own in looking after her children. But she belongs to a very active group of women campaigners and benefits from their practical support. Her need to find some form of support in combining care for her disabled son and single motherhood has been resolved through a women's network which would otherwise not have been of interest to her. It means that, for the first time in her life, she is now embedded in a wider social network, which gives her valuable experiences and self-esteem and has a stabilising influence on her situation.

In contrast, for Frau Alexander the process has not opened rewarding spheres of social contact. Frau Alexander is still quite isolated in her own home during the week; however, at weekends the whole family joins their biking community and they have a thriving social life. Her development lies in her having learned how to live fully with the potentially life-threatening condition of her son, wresting away the control of treatment and management from the medical profession. When it comes to her son's care, she has become a formidable negotiator and advocate, surpassing her own aspirations and wishes over time. She has never been interested in turning her competences into a public campaign, but she has managed to create a secure family context for her children, which is much more stable than was her own.

For Mrs Rajan, caring represents a process of personal and cultural change. As she did not receive the expected close, traditional family support, the birth of her second son is the catalyst for her to change. She now accepts outside assistance and help, and both partners now participate in domestic roles. Mr Rajan takes on household responsibilities, while Mrs Rajan has developed a life outside the home and participates actively in the multicultural community in East London.

Parallel lives

A third pattern of adaptation takes a middle ground between continuity and change. Carers in this category tend to switch between different biographical courses, which are often conflicting. Frau Blau and Frau Arndt, from East Germany, Mrs Buckley from London and Frau Hamann from West Germany are examples of this category. All are placed between conflicting adaptation patterns which offer different choices of how to address their new situation.

For most of them the caring trajectory is comparatively recent. Herr Blau had a stroke during the Wende time in 1991, in the middle of the disruptions to everyday life that followed unification. After the stroke, Frau Blau approached her caring as another work environment, by organising her husband's care and by campaigning for improved services for him. Some 18 months later, their personal conflicts were coming to the surface. The couple are increasingly isolated in their flat, throwing the partners together in a way they never were before. They have a different outlook on life. He prefers to remain at home and does not want to be left, while she craves outside contact. She feels unappreciated and over-burdened. As a consequence, the relationship between the couple is increasingly charged.

Frau Hamann also had a protracted period of settling down, including her son's initial illnesses and the uncertainties around their family circumstances during her husband's divorce. Her role as a full-time mother and carer is interrupted by her professional persona as a medical doctor. She is called upon by her colleagues, who treat her son and rely on her expertise in managing the disability. As we argued in the West German chapter, this presents her with a constant conflict of identity between herself as a mother and as a medical expert. As she perceives them as mutually exclusive spheres, as yet she has not been able to 'marry' these two identities, and this paralyses her ability to approach her own situation in a more active and positive way.

These renegotiations of carer identities are played out particularly poignantly in Mrs Buckley's case. During her daughter's childhood, she changed course a number of times, oscillating between an active and socially engaged lifestyle as part of a carer group when her daughter was young, and the more enclosed life with her daughter and her husband in recent years after Melanie's care needs changed. With Melanie growing up, falling back on family support and informal caring increasingly replaced the more independent approach the family initially took. With Melanie's impending adulthood and her husband's forthcoming retirement, Mrs

Buckley is again caught between the choice of independence for herself, her husband and Melanie, and maintaining her role as Melanie's sole carer. She agonises over Melanie's impending hysterectomy, which would offer the young woman freedom from gynaecological problems and the chance of a more independent life.

Mrs Buckley's example also indicates that the process of coming to terms with caring is not set in stone, but requires reorientation at different points. With Melanie's entering adulthood, her changing needs and physical development, the caring context has changed so that Mrs Buckley yet again has come to a biographical juncture which constitutes major biographical uncertainty. The caring trajectory is not a homogeneous process, but continually changes and requires different strategies and responses at different times.

Caring as struggle for identity

In many ways, the third group of carer adaptations (parallel lives) shows most acutely the personal struggle of finding a new identity as a carer. The relationship between Herr and Frau Blau has become so fragile, and her experience is so different from his, that they cannot even agree on their life before the stroke. As she struggles to come to terms with her own problems of dependency and loss of her former self, Frau Blau seems largely oblivious to the hurtful way she treats her husband.

The process mirrors that of coming to terms with chronic illness, as a biographical rupture which requires an active reworking of the self. Carers may experience periods of mourning over the life lost. They have to adjust to the new realities of life and, importantly, have to rework a personal sense of the future, a perspective of what is still possible in the context of this new life. Carers also have to come to terms with the changed 'otherness' of their partner, child or parent, and the changed relationships of dependency and interdependency. As the example of Frau Blau illustrates, it is not always a process that brings carer and cared-for person together: it can be emotionally isolating and can put relationships under intense strain.

Other carers have solved the inter-relational conflict: for the Grün family from East Germany, the challenge is met as a couple and later as a family trajectory in which all family members, including their son Jo, have a voice. One of the most dramatic indications of this in the interview account is the consistent use of 'we' in describing the experience of caring.

It is a means of drawing strength from the relational dimension of the experience without denying the personal aspect of caring.

For those carers in the continuity and change categories, the personal turmoil involved appears less acute. Carers have often worked through their anxiety, or have at least accommodated it. This can have its costs. Frau Alexander has never allowed herself to address the emotional trauma of the early years: during Andre's class trip, for instance, "I didn't know what to do with myself here, this calm, the emptiness somehow". While there is a lot of suppressed emotion in snippets of the account, hinting at unresolved feelings, overall, carers in the change category have found ways of reaching an emotional equilibrium in which emotional turmoil can be contained.

Frau Arndt manages to juggle her different roles as a single mother and carer of her son through a diverse informal support system which involves her parents, her friends near her own flat at weekends and a sophisticated self-help group. This complex set-up is part of a long-term plan to develop a more independent lifestyle. The determination and forward planning that go into achieving a more manageable working life and a higher income than before are new dimensions in Frau Arndt's life and are fuelled by the wish to take control of her and her son's life on her own terms. The process includes making compromises. At present, she is dependent on her own family for help with her son and has to accept a high degree of 'family' control over her movements and plans. And, although given the demands of her new job the situation is unlikely to change in the near future, with time Frau Arndt is likely to be able to achieve both her more independent life plans and a gradual merging of the two spheres of her life. Her strategy of 'holding out' is already showing some reward by the time of the second interview. Not only has she moved into a new flat with her son and has her new job, but her personal life is also more settled. She has closer contact with her former partner and they are spending more time as a family, thus reducing her dependency on her parents.

From trajectory to strategy

Openings and closures

As argued in the previous section, each of the patterns of biographical orientation can be a way of biographically coming to terms with caring, including the emotional and inter-relational changes they imply. In the case of those carers who integrate caring into their current lives, this can be an empowering strategy of coping with the new situation, particularly at the beginning of the caring process. Frau Jakob's strategy of seeing her caring as an extension of her family loyalty and kin obligation enables her to take charge of the situation by discharging her husband from hospital and taking on his care, regardless of the difficulties. Similarly, Frau Schumann's insistence on keeping her son at home provides her with a framework for her family life in which her son can participate. And given that Herr Speyer's married relationship is based around his wife's dependency on him, her deteriorating condition does not fundamentally change their relationship. As a strategy, being able to fall back on some sort of continuum very often provides a necessary equilibrium at a time of great upheaval.

The insistence of Frau Hegemann that "we are a normal family" is emblematic of the need to maintain normality and continuity in the face of the disruption and turmoil created by the onset of the illness:

> Our family life carried on, obviously with some constrictions, that is clear. But my husband was never the type to despair, and therefore it wasn't too difficult for myself.

However, as a coping strategy over time, continuing in this mould becomes risky and harder to sustain, particularly since the context changes. With Herr Hegemann's increasing dependency and physical isolation at home and with the children growing up, it becomes harder for Frau Hegemann to maintain the normal family life routine upheld for so many years. Her double role of breadwinner and homemaker is barely sustainable for the family, and the children are rebelling in different ways against the status quo.

With the increasing dependency of the disabled person, carers are pulled into the routine of caring, without a strategy to reassess the situation or to change arrangements. Carers of disabled children in particular find it difficult to make plans for the changing circumstances when their children grow up. Making the 'jump' to let their children lead lives that are more independent is sometimes impossible in a context where so much of the carer's identity is bound up with the home environment. Peter Bally's continued living at home is the classic example of this. Although Mrs Bally and Frau Schumann realise that their current lifestyles are no longer the appropriate setting for their children, they find it difficult to develop other solutions or to accept guidance from outside.

—

One potential consequence is the resentment that can be bred in the carer and the subsequent deterioration in the caring relationship. Mr and Mrs Rushton bicker over the practicalities of the caring routine. Mrs Rushton feels so pressured by her caring responsibilities that even the services they receive increase her feelings of being burdened. Mr Rushton's attendance at the day centre is preceded by a flurry of activity: "I have been seeing to his enemas. I've been feeding him, I've been washing him".

The problem for these carers in the longer term is the fact that they have no alternative strategies to fall back on. At the outset of the caring process, the continuity of a previous life theme offers stability and a point of orientation and control over the context of caring. Within the caring relationship, it may also offer a starting point for maintaining the relationship. Over the longer term, however, the lack of alternatives creates a situation which can easily become oppressive to either carer or disabled person or both.

For those carers who develop new identities or for whom caring means a departure from their life course, the initial period can be traumatic. Frau Grün's expression "… and then we were on our own, on empty fields …" conveys something of the stress and loneliness felt by the couple at this time. Frau Alexander is more candid: "… one has problems oneself … and these people [nurses etc] are not normally there for that … everything to do with yourself you have to sort out yourself".

The cost of the initial trauma and the process of adaptation sometimes breaks relationships. Frau Meissner's and Frau Arndt's partners left in the aftermath of the birth of their children. Facing this process successfully as a couple can strengthen the relationship: Frau Grün acknowledges that the support between the couple is a crucial ingredient for developing a strategy:

> If you want to look for something positive in this it would be that, then perhaps that it, well, that the task brings you closer together. I think it makes it a lot easier, because there are always problems.

Caring can open the way for forging new identities, and can also open up new spheres of activities. For the Mertons, caring is bound up with their identities as a disabled couple. Care in Mr Merton's terms is both a labour of love and an act of political solidarity with people who need assistance. The Mahlers in West Germany also shift the framework of care services and caring onto new ground, securing the support of all of their family, as well as colleagues and friends.

While there is little doubt that the initial trauma of a change strategy can be immense, as a strategy for coping with the caring task on a longer-term basis, it appears more sustainable. Building a new identity and success in improving services or personal circumstances constitute a powerful personal carer identity and a basis for facing new external challenges with confidence. In particular, a change strategy provides an orientation to the future, which makes strategic planning and agency a real prospect. The Alexanders have adapted their lifestyles a number of times to accommodate their son's changing needs, using the resources available to them in imaginative ways, including the ingenious idea of buying the camper van, which gives the family so much freedom to travel. Frau Meissner's role as an informal carer has effectively finished with her daughter going off to do further training at college and living independently. However, this has not been a traumatic separation, but is regarded by mother and daughter as a development. Frau Meissner is still involved in her daughter's life, and they go on holidays together, but the relationship has moved on. They both have their separate identities now, and different arenas of activities. Frau Meissner has her own role as a voluntary disability advisor and her activities have spread beyond the realm of her daughter's needs.

For the East German carers, the transitional nature of the Wende context poses a unique problem for adaptation. As one system is supplanting another, they also have to cope with the unhinging of their life worlds and the discontinuity of welfare systems. It is not surprising that the strategies of 'new' East German carers are intrinsically linked to the Wende situation itself. For Frau Arndt and Frau Blau, the experience of caring is synonymous with the external upheavals; personal dimensions and traumas are even overshadowed by the 'larger' events. The repercussions of this are visible in the Blau case. Frau Blau's struggles with the authorities and her anger at the uncaring bureaucracy of the 'West' German system hide the emotional turmoil of her personal situation. The Arndts' criticism of the system equally diverts attention from the tensions and conflicts in their households. Much of their account is directed at the inadequacies of the system, while the personal dimension remains muted. Clearly, over the longer term these carers need to separate out the subjective and objective dimensions of their situations in order to achieve personal stability.

For the longer-standing carers, the upheavals of the Wende have been largely contained within their established strategies. However, the Grüns' increasing worry and self-interrogation about the extent of their son's disabilities, hinted at near the end of the interview, may mark a tentative change to the strategy of 'normalisation' which has dominated their approach for a number of years. For them, the new system offers the chance to move on.

Negotiating support

As caring strategies, continuity and change also have repercussions for the way in which support can be drawn into the caring context. The notions of home and family are a constant theme in all the adaptation strategies, and carers are committed to sustaining their caring roles. However, carers who have chosen to build their caring strategies on biographical continuity are often doing this from within the home sphere, while those who have opted for biographical change tend to be more oriented towards the outside world.

Carers in the continuity group have fewer services and in many cases services are less welcome. For Mrs Rushton and Frau Hegemann, linking up with the outside world is felt as an additional burden. Mrs Rushton resents the extra work and the infringement of her private sphere caused by the different services which are organised into her home to assist her husband. She has to wait for the night nurses to put her husband to bed, and she has to rush to get her husband ready for the ambulance. Frau Hegemann is tired of the role she is obliged to play in the local MS group – in her view a futile exercise which she only continues out of loyalty to her husband's past role in it. Both women have experience of services for their husbands, and their cynicism expresses an ambivalence concerning threats to their privacy. They are keeping services at arms' length.

Frau Jakob and Herr Speyer even more actively refuse services which would intrude into their private spheres of home. Neither carer has been able to absorb the shift in family structures and each still harks back to an ideology of traditional family life which is no longer a viable option in either East or West Germany. As their identities are so bound up with the privacy of the home, they cannot contemplate outside assistance to any degree.

All these carers' identification with the home sphere coincides with and reinforces a reluctance to draw in or engage with outside services, whether these be informal contacts or formal services. As carers hold on to former identities and previous lives through the caring process, the division between public and private deepens and it becomes increasingly difficult to negotiate services actively. As such, they tend to be in the best instance passive recipients of services. In many of the cases, they only seem to receive a minimum of services and no social support.

Alternatives to this mode of passivity in organising support are illustrated by Frau Luchtig and Mr Allahm. While Frau Luchtig sees herself as a lifelong carer, her mother's caring needs are as yet limited. Nevertheless, Frau Luchtig has managed to mobilise considerable informal support among her acquaintances. Her ingenious device of inviting a group of people for the afternoon is a tribute to her skill in managing the different threads in her life. Mr Allahm, who combines a very active life with the role of caring for his wife, also manages to gather an effective informal support network, in addition to an extensively negotiated service package. In both cases, the public engagement and the balancing of private family enclosure and public activity are long-practised features of their life course, a resource that is not easily available to other carers.

More often, active negotiation is the consequence of having fought for services and part of a traumatic learning curve. Frau Meissner had to take on the education authorities to have her daughter participate in normal schooling. This experience set her on a route of regular campaigning for disability issues and into wider social engagement. The process was not so much planned as something that "happened", as she puts it. In terms of her private life, her resistance to public authority has liberated the family from some constraining conventions. She and her daughter have regular and close contact with her ex-husband and his new family, a constellation that is commented on by observing neighbours. For Mr Merton, the path of campaigning was opened through his wife's contacts with the disability lobby. Interestingly, he has turned this political connection to social use and community action. In assisting a series of people in his neighbourhood, Mr Merton not only traverses what are often politically separate types of disability and dependency, but also balances political commitment with social engagement in his community.

Frau Mahler and Frau Alexander redefine the boundaries of public and private in their negotiation with service providers. They negotiate a maximum of services and employ them in innovative and individual strategies. They combine the interests of their families with those of the cared-for person. Together with another couple, who are also fostering a child with healthcare problems, the Mahlers are planning to build a house, so that the children can grow up in a protected and rural environment. They will be able to finance this through the income from fostering

Stella. Frau Alexander also takes calculated risks in her care for her son in order to bring about service provision and to maintain control over the caring situation, challenging welfare and health professionals in the process. In both cases, the strategies of these carers dispute and stretch the boundaries of service providers on a continuous basis.

Outward orientation and biographical change are closely linked processes. It is the experience of engaging with the outside world, with professionals, with the system of welfare, which opens the possibility of change in the first place. It may also be that this tendency is particularly prevalent among younger parents of children with disabilities, where attitudes are more open and life patterns less firmly established. However, as the cases of Frau Schumann and Frau Hamann show, this is not always the case. One additional factor that seems to propel individuals into becoming more active in negotiating care is the degree of reflexivity about their situation, which seems to facilitate change. Initially, Frau Alexander's path was certainly an instinctive reaction to the appalling prospect of long-term hospital care. However, over time and with an increasing record of 'victories' over officialdom, her ability to act purposefully and strategically has increased. In the case of the Grüns, the process is much more deliberate from the start. Supported by a wide church network, they can tap into it for information and support, and early on make decisions about the treatment they want to pursue for their son's development.

Lessons for intervention

We have argued that those carers with an outward, active orientation are best placed to respond dynamically to the caring process and to sustain caring over the longer term. This group also demonstrates something about the creativity which the private sphere of welfare is able to generate. These carers transform the formal system of provision and achieve greater equality with professionals. On a practical level, they develop skills of negotiation, organise external support and operate successfully in different contexts. Personally, they emerge as flexible and independent agents, capable of structuring the caring process over the long term and managing crisis successfully. Nurturing and supporting this ability may be a way forward for a practice of service intervention which recognises the agency and autonomy of carers in shaping their own situation.

The analysis of carer strategies points to the complex way in which welfare identities are constructed and developed. It also highlights the paradox that reflexivity and self-knowledge do not necessarily enhance agency and strategic action. Carers such as Frau Luchtig and Frau Hamann are quite aware of the limitations of their current situations, although this knowledge does not 'free' them to make changes. In contrast, carers such as Frau Alexander and Frau Meissner, who have made large strides in self-development, are not particularly reflective about their own situations. It seems that reflexivity (Giddens, 1991) on its own is not enough and is not always necessary to engender transformative action, at least in the field of informal care.

In terms of intervention, the biographical approach also fits into debates concerning new social work practice, stressing the significance of grounding intervention in everyday experience and taking seriously the differential subjectivities and capacities of welfare subjects (Williams, 1993; Cooper, 1999; Shanin, 1998). As indicated in chapter two, the research findings of Baldock and Ungerson (1994) also support the need for policies and administrative systems to be sensitive to life-course and everyday experiences of client groups.

It is in this applied use of biographical approaches to caring that notions of strategy and continuity and change may provide an alternative approach to supporting informal carers. Changes that may affect current caring routines and strategies may be sparked by personal developments or external contingencies, such as the development of the illness, and changes in life circumstances and relationships. Even the most well-adjusted caring situations hold the potential for crisis. At the same time, caring strategies which embrace values of negotiation and social engagement and preserve horizons of change constitute a resilient form of informal care. Services which take the biographical context of caring into account should consider how strategies develop, how services relate to personal development, and the timing of interventions. We conclude this chapter with a discussion of these points.

Developing a caring strategy

One of the paradoxes of an outward mode of caring is that it is at least partly born out of the (often antagonistic) relationship with formal service provision. Carers such as Frau Alexander, the Grün family and Mr Merton have achieved their current strategies because of the inadequacy of services and provision. Becoming a fighter is in a way part of the process of developing more independence. An important driving force in Frau

Alexander's pursuit of services was the fact that health services and social services did not envisage her son Andre being looked after at home. Similarly, the Grüns' rejection of the system allowed them to develop their own personal routes to services. For these carers, the shortcomings of the formal provision itself contributed significantly to the development of their caring strategies.

But this process has a high personal cost. Frau Grün's and Frau Alexander's muted comments about the early lives of their children, and Mr Merton's silence about the time after he was diagnosed with epilepsy, make reference to the difficult process of adaptation to disability and caring, and hint at the personal pain and trauma experienced. While experiences of resistance and of individual and collective action can be a source of empowerment and agency, carers also need to be supported through the difficult period of trauma and adjustment. In terms of services, there is a balance to be struck between the need for appropriate services and a practice of fostering independence among carers.

Services and personal development

Our analysis flags up the need for an approach to service provision which strikes a balance between adequate practical services and more person-centred support. It is interesting to note the role in carers' accounts in all three societies of significant social work professionals (often at quite low levels of the hierarchy) and the importance of social networks. Frau Planck mentions the intervention of her social worker in introducing her to the community women's group as a turning point in her situation. As the case of Mrs Rajan shows, the sensitive intervention of sympathetic professionals can encourage personal development. Such contacts, together with the opportunity to participate in local networks, are vital links to the outside world.

The timing of interventions

Support in the past might have allowed carers such as Frau Jakob, Herr Speyer or Mrs Rushton to come to terms with the changing contexts of their lives. Frau Jakob only had limited advice from the hospital about caring tasks, following her husband's stroke. Her husband's care needs neither fitted with her understanding of family obligations, nor provided her with personally appropriate choices. Mrs Rushton only seems to have received technical advice, without regard to her personal circumstances or sensitivities. Jones and Rupp (2000) argue that Mrs Rajan could have benefited earlier from sympathetic and culturally sensitive intervention.

Even in the more dynamic strategies, service provision plays an important structuring role in facilitating or constraining development and change. There are windows of opportunity during the caring process where intervention may engender change and carers can begin a process of adjustment. Developmental social work already points to periods of receptiveness for intervention. Identifying these moments may pose the strongest challenge to an intervention practice which takes the biographical dimension of caring into account. Such an approach implies that the framework of support needs to be sensitised to periods of transition and change. A crucial time for intervention may be in the early phases of the caring process, when strategies are still open to modification. In particular, supporting carers in moving between different kinds of adaptation might enable them to adopt more open strategies.

SIX

Carers and the social world

Our study demonstrates that carers' orientations and dispositions towards the public, social and private spheres and their ways of negotiating among them cannot be read off from formal welfare systems (Chamberlayne, 1993). Carers' practices in everyday situations are to a large extent structurally determined, yet they are often considerably at odds with institutionalised policies. In this chapter we explore this paradox. We ask what energises creative responses in carers, what features of informal social structures which are contiguous with carers' lives enable them to negotiate and access outside support, and what cultural dynamics leave them torn between home and non-home identities and resources, or even cause them to retreat into a strategy of isolation.

A key concern is to distinguish the ingredients of social infrastructures which propel carers into greater outer-connectedness and prevent them from becoming enclosed in a narrow world of domesticity. We are also interested in the extent to which these ingredients are in fact the focus of social interventions in Germany and Britain, and whether they figure in contemporary debates concerning social practice and the future of social policy. In our view, carers who negotiate wider connections and for whom caring becomes a process of personal and social development, model the 'active welfare subject' which social policy purports to be in search of. It would be all too easy to attribute the outward propulsion of some carers to their individual personalities and so blame others who remain more rooted in the home. Our purpose, however, is to focus on and distinguish key elements of the *structural dynamics* which give rise to proactive and outwardly oriented strategies in caring, and to discuss what kinds of social policy interventions might support such social engagement. In doing so we are aided by the comparative method, which brings these structural features into view.

In order to intervene at the level of the informal sphere, social policy needs a language and understanding of socio-cultural processes. One of the sources of our own rather tentative terminology is Riley's (1988) notion of the social, which she defines as a fluid sphere of communal interaction and public health reform adjacent to the home, which has often provided avenues to wider public involvement, but which political science has continually fenced off as not 'political'[1]. Anthropology, by contrast, recognises that exchanges in intermediate networks and sociability often hold the key to power relations in wider society (Hann and Dunn, 1996). Recent social policy attention to informal social structures and relations as empowering resources for individuals and communities lies close to this kind of thinking. However, it is important to distinguish the political agendas which underlie concerns to strengthen social capital. Referring to the field of education, Gamarnikow and Green (1999) contrast the conventional norms which inspire Third Way communitarianism with a more radical and participatory approach to civic engagement. In seeking to differentiate the implications for professionals of encouraging wider social engagement, we have found it useful to contrast the individualised 'rights' orientation within empowerment thinking in Britain with the more 'relational' approach of continental thinking towards citizenship and community development work in Germany (Donati, 1995).

This chapter is in three sections. The first characterises the cultural dynamics of caring by comparing the features of home- and outward-oriented as well as 'torn' cases in the three societies, and the different push and pull factors underlying carers' orientations to the public and private spheres. The second moves across and beyond the three societies to identify key features of social infrastructures which make the outside world accessible to carers. The purpose here is to identify aspects of the dynamics of informal cultures into which interventions could be made, in order to foster and broaden social engagement, including among the most domestically confined. The third section examines the extent to which debates concerning community care, social practice and the Third Way in Germany and Britain already incorporate such orientations, and whether current service structures are able to realise the active model of welfare.

Carers' relationships with the social world

In our study, we found that the interplay of personal factors, family pressures and service contexts producing a particular orientation to the home or the outside world was quite different in each society. So were the individual motivations for each strategy. Differences in motivation and in determining pressures resulted in quite different forms of public,

Figure I: The caring triangle

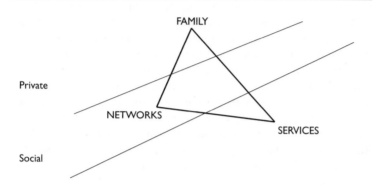

Private

FAMILY

NETWORKS

SERVICES

Social

Public

social and private engagement, and therefore in constituting relationships between the three arenas.

We have often found it helpful to think in terms of a caring triangle, in which the three points of focus may vary for different purposes. The caring triangle which we used initially in comparing cases incorporated the contingency of the disability; family and personal dynamics; and the public world, including employment, services and associational life. In this chapter, in order to keep a central focus on the informal sphere, we focus on the relationship between family, networks and services which forms the crucial triangle (see Figure 1). Employment, which is another important dimension, is kept to the margins of this particular discussion.

Why is it that in West Germany and Britain the outwardly-oriented carers seemed somewhat exceptional to each society's central dynamic, while in East Germany they epitomised the system? For the difference between outward-orientedness and domestic entrapment is rich in social significance. Outward-orientedness is associated with social vibrancy and creativity. It gives rise to widely transferable social competences and to equality between professionals and carers as lay experts, and it contributes to the density of social trust and social capital, enabling carers to be more resourceful in seeking out tailor-made support. The more differentiated the solutions, the more diversified the social fabric and the resources and opportunities for others. Entrapment, by contrast, reduces carers' resourcefulness and perceptions of alternative solutions, diminishing their energy, their adaptability and their capacity to be proactive.

However much modernisation may in other respects have changed relations between public and private spheres, West Germany and Britain have maintained a considerable degree of domestic confinement for many women carers, together with a gendered sense of vocation in the home (Blinkert and Klie, 1999). West German carers in our study were more likely to have been full-time housewives or to entertain the idea of that as a fulfilling role, and to be subject to family expectations of that kind. It was as if they were fenced into the private sphere, and in order to have a strong outward orientation they needed to either be positioned outside the traditional family form, or to exercise great strength of will. In Britain, carers seemed to have more outside connections, especially when children were young, and to experience a weaker cultural pull of the family. They were more likely to work or have worked outside the home, at least part-time. Nevertheless, when services failed and in the absence of professional encouragement, they tended to lapse back into thinking 'family is best'. Partner support in caring (usually by husbands), which may have been strong in the past, would tend to wane as home-centredness set in. And the carers' groups which we encountered seemed to endorse the isolated conditions of home-based caring, rather than leading on to wider social connectedness and personal development.

In East Germany, the family barrier and the sense of personal vocation in the home had been removed by three generations of mothers' outside employment. East German carers were less enclosed in a world of caring, with no official expectations of home-based caring, a vigorous culture of seeking solutions through informal networking and a pattern of ready support from certain professionals. This produced considerable continuity between strategies used in everyday life-world situations and those required to find support for caring, whereas in West Germany and Britain there was a more dislocated situation. Loose networking in East Germany and the social trust which permeated it (see Chapter Three) meant that carers were likely to make the connections they needed to meet a particular situation, and to develop their own knowledge and competences in the process of seeking help and challenging the authorities.

We now examine this generalised pattern of findings in more detail, by comparing the dynamics underlying home, torn and outward orientations in each of the three societies. Figure 2 lists the case studies we are considering under these headings.

Figure 2: List of detailed case studies

	Home-oriented	'Torn' cases	Outwardly-oriented
West Germany	Jakob/Hamann	Luchtig/Hegemann	Mahler/Alexander
	'Trapped in the private sphere'	'Painful compromises'	'Working the system'
East Germany	Speyer	Blau/Arndt	Meissner/Grün
	'Retreat into the private sphere'	'Transition cases'	'Trawling the social sphere'
Britain	Buckley/Rushton	Rajan/Bally	Allahm/Merton
	'Family is best'	'Reluctant transitions'	'Creating the social'

Home-oriented cases

The nature of commitment among the home-oriented cases varies considerably. The 'trapped' situation of the two West German carers has involved purposeful decisions. However, while Frau Jakob has acted on and maintains a strong personal belief in home caring, Frau Hamann has been caught in a contradictory fantasy of personal fulfilment, and bitterly regrets her situation. The other three carers in East Germany and Britain are repelled by the public sphere more than pulled into the home. Herr Speyer's fortress mentality largely derives from rebellion against the public sphere, Mrs Rushton is concerned to guard the privacy of her home from outside intrusion, and Mrs Buckley has lapsed back into the private sphere because of a weakening of outside support.

Frau Jakob made the active decision to bring her very ill husband back home, and Frau Hamann a similar one to abandon her career, family and friends to make a family life with a divorcing man in a family practice. Both have been strongly pulled by traditional family ideology, both are denied wider family support, and neither has outside connections. Frau Jakob is personally and inflexibly committed to family caring and is bitterly disappointed in the isolation it brings her. She has not grasped the shift in family and social structures which has taken place in her own lifetime. Nor is her philosophy, which is espoused by public ideology, any longer consistent with social reality. Frau Hamann has been impelled to her marriage by some inner need or fantasy of domestic fulfilment, which may well be fed by tradition. But it is not a belief to which she is overtly committed. Curiously, her own mother had similarly sacrificed her career as an artist to marriage. A woman of Frau Hamann's education and experience of West German society might be expected to have anticipated the hostile and restrictive family culture and structure she has chosen to enter. But the situation has closed around her rather than being of her own making. For both these carers, the dynamic is one of pull into the family sphere.

While Herr Speyer's actions have much in common with Frau Jakob's, and the two carers are of the same generation, he seems to be motivated more by rebellion against the public sphere than by the pull of home life. Just as his decision to buy into his wife's family's taxi business was a repudiation of East German collectivist norms, so his individualist solution of dedicating his life to care of his wife is a repudiation of socialist public policy. The available forms of public provision are undoubtedly of a poor standard, but he has not even begun to explore the possibilities and has actively walled himself off from outside support. At least, that is his own definition of his situation and of his identity. In fact, he seems to have considerable support from both his daughters, with whom he and his wife have stayed for months at a time, and he also has moral support from and ready accessibility to a woman doctor and a community nurse, even though he rejects their advice.

The relationship of Mrs Rushton and Mrs Buckley (British cases) to the private and public spheres lies between these two extremes. They are neither particularly pulled towards the home sphere nor repelled by public services. Instead, absence of personal support, whether professional or informal, and the poor quality of services are determining factors in their situations. In rejecting the option of more domiciliary help, Mrs Rushton is avoiding an invasion of both time and space; she dislikes strangers coming into her bedroom, and also dislikes having to adapt to other people's time schedules and unreliability. In guarding her privacy, she may also be keeping hidden her conflictual relationship with her husband. Mrs Buckley's turn to family care derives from the historic worsening of public services. In Melanie's childhood, when Mrs Buckley was helped by hospital personnel to resume employment, she did so, but she has no such firm guidance in the shift to adult independent living for Melanie. In giving up work she is impelled by the gap between children's and adult services in Britain, and by gender taboos attendant on her daughter's maturity and gynaecological problems, which exclude Mr Buckley from much direct caring. The more she takes on Melanie's full care, the more she feels indispensable, and wider friendships become replaced by a smaller carer circle.

'Torn' cases

The torn cases are either pulled between clashing dependencies or being forced to make unwilling personal transitions. The same patterns emerge in this category as among the home-oriented cases, of home pull in the case of West Germany and of outward push in the case of East Germany, with Britain in between.

The two West German cases, despite having outside links, are unable to surmount the pull of traditional ideologies and structures of West German family life. Frau Hegemann is predominantly passive, showing little sign of enjoying an independent identity as breadwinner, and only reluctantly attending the multiple sclerosis group which her husband and she established. Home pressures seem to paralyse her, with young adult children and her husband making demands which are difficult to reconcile. Frau Luchtig is in a much more active process of struggle over her identity, seizing every opportunity to develop her independent craft and musical interests. Yet her lifetime of turbulent subordination to her mother in the family grocery continues, and she dreads her mother becoming more ill and her husband more demanding on retirement. Outside help is being offered – even pushed – by the professionals, but is not taken because of her mother's refusal.

The two East German cases are caught between the pressures of traditional family forms and structurally supported impulses to make outward connections. The outward pull from the East German model of full employment for women is intensified by the challenge of unification. The mission of saving Frau Arndt's family from social assistance fortifies her father's patriarchal tendencies and makes her feel trapped with her family during the week. The family's facilitation of her training impels her towards independence, however, as do her links with a particularly effective self-help group. Frau Blau also, far from submitting to a role as pensioner housewife and carer, continually turns to the outside world, drawing on her employment skills to do daily battle for equipment, benefits, cures and holidays, and going out for walks and to the garden. While she experiences the lead role in public as a challenge and feels guilty at leaving her husband for any period of time, she is actively reflecting on these issues and rather proudly undergoing a process of personal change.

The British cases once again show the crucial role of services, especially at transitional life stages. Mrs Rajan has been coming into greater contact with outside support, while Mrs Bally has been disengaging from her previous networks. However, Mrs Bally's own old age is compelling her to consider full outside support for her son Peter. In Mrs Rajan's case, rather than any positive pull of family culture or ideology, it was the shame of disability, lack of trust in the outside world, and failure of the welfare professions to intervene which for many years locked her into a private sphere of helplessness and hopelessness. Only with the entry of professionals, starting with the birth of a second son, did she become open to outside support and begin a process of development. Her life change parallels shifts in the public sphere, from the earlier racism of public services to the later multiculturalism of her borough. Mrs Bally, by contrast, used to be proactive in the public sphere, moving house to achieve integrated nursery care and schooling for her son, and using extensive networks for respite care. Helped by her nursing training, she has used Peter's care, just as she used the care of her mother over many years, as a central formation of family life. Thus for 20 years or so, she actively held her public and private identities and commitments in balance. But then, starting with Peter's transition from adequate educational to inadequate adult services, her home orientation comes to dominate. She loses her outside connections, she fails to connect with positive provision for independent living, and Peter's development recedes.

Despite the diversity of orientations among the torn cases, clear patterns emerge in each society. While Frau Hegemann is rather passively suspended between her public and private roles, Frau Luchtig is constantly struggling to be freer of her mother's claims on her and to have more access to the outside world. Yet both these West German women are stuck, with few signs of personal change. The East German women, Frau Arndt and Frau Blau, more strongly based in and pulled towards the public sphere, are undergoing personal transitions – Frau Arndt in her education and social experience, Frau Blau, more reflectively, in her marriage relationship. The reorientation towards more outside forms of support in the British cases, Mrs Rajan and Mrs Bally, is not so much self-willed as the result of confrontations between conflicting responsibilities. For Mrs Rajan at least, the result is an increasingly valued personal transition.

Outwardly-oriented cases

The outwardly-oriented cases share an ease in bridging public and private spheres, although the routes to this balance are different in the three societies. Whereas in West Germany the balance seems to derive from coming into contact with an alternative kind of lifestyle, in East Germany it is part and parcel of everyday strategies in the wider society. Among the British cases, the bridging of public and private spheres is a gendered phenomenon, based on transposing former (male) occupational and life skills to particular caring situations, although some of the women carers have bridged public and private spheres in the past.

In West Germany, it seems to be a freedom from traditional family structures and ideologies which allows the Mahlers and Frau Alexander to 'work the system', exploiting the relative generosity of West German benefits in order to achieve mobility and flexibility in conducting their lives. In the case of the Mahlers, personal and public lifestyles are so closely interlinked that family privacy is simply not an operative concept. For both families, the private sphere is friendship centred, which creates permeability between the public and private spheres.

In East Germany, outwardly-oriented strategies of 'trawling the social sphere' conform with the general cultural pattern of working through informal networks to procure the necessities of everyday life, and with the self-evidence that women should work and anchor an identity in the public world beyond the home. Frau Meissner fought for years to keep her daughter Katrin out of institutional care. Later, resisting her designation to a vocational school in Berlin which would remove her from their orbit of support and yield low-level qualifications, the Meissners negotiated a solution in Leipzig, managing the transport around their two full-time jobs over a two-year period. Likewise, by means of networking and huge physical effort, the Grüns have achieved integrated schooling and much greater mobility for their son Jo than might have been expected. For both families, networking has included help from professionals who implicitly share the same humanist counterculture of opposition to the official system. Privacy is a key issue for the Grüns, who are carefully guarded in their management of outside relationships. Frau Meissner, whose dedication to Katrin is at the cost of her own personal relationships, finds great personal fulfilment in her social activities and contacts. Both parents and professionals are also propelled in their efforts by policies and structures which greatly favour the less disabled as compared with the more severely immobilised.

The exceptional ease of access to the public sphere of the two British outward-orientated carers is because they are men. It is the cultural norm for men to have identities anchored in the public sphere – a situation which otherwise in our study only pertained among the East German women carers. British researchers have observed that men carers organise caring as 'work' (Ungerson, 1987, p 104), which could also imply a greater readiness to involve others. Mr Allahm's strategy of founding a church fulfils his search for emotional support and provides a supply of helpers for his wife. This creates a fluidity between public and private spheres and solves his spiritual needs, which are intensified by the loss of closeness with his wife. By marrying a disability activist, Mr Merton enters the worlds of disability and caring politics, which leads to more and more campaigning and advice work. This transposes his earlier physical activism as a seaman, and his former 'caring' identity as a lifeguard, into skills as a carer. Staving off the debilitating effects of his own epilepsy through this mutually sustaining marriage, Mr Merton's problem becomes one of preserving his private space from total invasion – he has to lock himself in his room with the telephone off to get an hour's peace.

From this richly varied patchwork we can make some general observations on the bearing of the social sphere on carers' motivations and states of feeling. Among our interviewees there is a remarkable lack of positive commitment to a home-centred identity. Perhaps only Frau Jakob has positively chosen and would actively maintain such a role, and even she finds herself feeling greatly oppressed by her isolation and the failure of her imagined wider family support. Frau Hamann's fantasy of personal fulfilment in a domestic setting has rapidly collapsed, irrespective of having a disabled child. Rather than exhibiting a positive pull to home-centredness, carers seem more likely to adopt that strategy because of hostility to or fear of the public sphere, or because of the failure of outside services, or because of a waning of support to maintain bridges between private and public worlds. Keeping up links with the outside world requires enormous energy. Frau Luchtig exhausts herself in an unsuccessful struggle against the demands of her mother, but carers who are more supported in their outward orientation seemed energised, not least by the personal development which their outside connections bring them.

We now go on to examine in more detail the nature of the supports which seem necessary to maintaining an outward orientation. This will help us to highlight what our data contribute to social policy understanding of the dynamics of the informal sphere.

Fostering features of the informal sphere

A key characteristic of the outwardly oriented carers is their ready ability to bridge public and private worlds. For the home-oriented carers, the outside world lacks this accessibility. This may be because these carers are structurally and emotionally pulled into the home sphere, because outside services seem dubious, because the outside world feels inhospitable, or because they lack mediating connections through professionals or networks.

Caring situations are structured by a combination of factors rather than by single determinants. Employment does not guarantee continued connection with the outside world, any more than poor services inevitably propel carers towards home-based solutions. We need to consider factors in relation to each other and to hold dimensions of gender constantly in mind.

From the complex matrix of structural features we have identified we can distinguish three kinds of conditions which favour outward-connectedness: activity routes, shared cultures and personal support. Carers can find a route out of domestic confinement into the outside world in a range of practical activities, employment, informal networks and engagement in welfare or community services. These ways of moving between public and private worlds are highly gendered, and critical in structuring identities and caring strategies, for both men and women. It seems that the common culture will ideally be a counterculture, involving personal relationships, trust and a sense of being fortified by sharing in a common culture. A sense of being personally supported is also a crucial resource, whether through a marriage partnership or by a professional whom one likes. This support may be moral as much as practical, and will involve a sense of interdependence based on some kind of equality. Bridging public, social and private worlds seems to involve a combined sense of 'belonging', control and autonomy. This combination generates the confidence to act and take initiatives and to challenge authority, and brings great energy – the energy of the more outwardly oriented carers is phenomenal.

Activity routes

Employment identity

According to classical socialism, employment is crucial in rescuing women from the confines of domesticity. Through employment, women gain a public and class identity and access to organised politics. In our study, an employment history and identity seems critical in predisposing carers to orient to the outside world. Patterns of female employment in the three societies run parallel with the greater home-orientedness in West Germany and outward-orientedness in East Germany, with Britain in between. The 'torn' East German carers (Frau Arndt and Frau Blau), either of whom might have lapsed into home-centredness in equivalent circumstances in West Germany or Britain, are propelled by their respective expectations and habits of work to look for outside resources and solutions. Male identities, in which employment is central, seem responsible for the easier bridging of public and private spheres by the two outwardly-oriented British carers. Mrs Buckley, who has formerly been more outwardly-oriented, was fully employed in her earlier caring career.

We saw how the British pattern of part-time work gives carers more outside contact than non-working housewives have, but of an indeterminate kind. Professional and part-time work could be a way of managing the home situation rather than a means of building outside connections. Mrs Bally uses her nursing work outside and inside the home to this end; Frau Hamann's medical qualifications increase her in-laws' expectations of her coping capacities and thereby her isolation. Frau Hegemann's home-based concerns and identity leave her unaffected by outside connections, although the low quality of her employment may be a detracting factor.

Employment by no means guarantees the East German kind of outward propulsion – it can be heavily mitigated by family structures and gendered identities and expectations concerning caring. Professional skills, which may facilitate the bridging of public and private worlds, can also lock a carer into isolated self-sufficiency, as we saw with Frau Hamann. On the other hand, an employment-derived outward orientation may be shored up by a culture of networking.

Networks

Among our case studies we find at least three different forms of networking. One involves an ongoing flow of strangers, the second a more closed-in group, and the third a flexible but tailor-made network.

The first type of network is a loose impersonal form in which people have the confidence to approach strangers for information or help. Their confidence probably lies in knowing that others beneficially do the same thing. They themselves have made such approaches before and habitually do so. This pattern of informal social relations permeated East German society, and seems common in Britain among parents of young children. It is the loose, horizontal form of networking which Putnam (1993), in his study of northern Italy, associates with flexible cooperation and trust, the mobilising of social capital, and the fostering of civic competence. Such social relationships lead further outwards, beyond a tight sphere of acquaintances. Their fluidity means that almost any problem can be solved – somewhere out there someone will have the answer. In working this human version of the web system, other viewpoints will be encountered, and networking thus becomes a developmental process. It is typified in classical sociology as Gesellschaft society, in which people associate with each other according to their individual needs and freely chosen interests. The contrasting form is Gemeinschaft society based on traditional families and communities, in which roles are prescribed (Tönnies, 1955; Rosanvallon, 1988, p 207).

The carer groups in which so many of the British carers participated are a more enclosed form of network, in which relationships do not extend outwards. Set up by professionals for formal purposes of consultation as well as mutual support, the groups have a specific membership – there is no wider meeting of strangers in the process of formation. Although more organised than loose networks, and bearing a publicly recognised status, their function is quite narrow: to bolster home-centred caring. In this sense they may represent little more than an extension of the private sphere (Williams, 1993). Gaining advice and mutual sympathy helps in tolerating burdensome situations, as does 'having a laugh', but does not challenge the traditional parameters of family care, or mobilise wider social resources in its support. As we have indicated in the British chapter (Chapter Four), this type of carer group has become incorporated, losing the political independence and new social movement features which the disability movement retains (Gordon and Donald, 1993; Barnes, 1997; Campbell and Oliver, 1997).

The third type of network is both more individually or tailor-made and more impersonal. While its setting up involves organisational competence and personal initiative in meeting strangers, and its membership may be flexibly open, it is formed for a specific local and even individual purpose. This is how we characterise the church organisation set up by Mr Allahm and the advocacy work which Mr Merton undertakes. In both cases, the activities seem to hinge on their personalities and will live and die with them. Frau Hager, depicted at the very beginning of the book, is another example of such networking. Although severely tied to home by her own disabilities and by caring for her blind and bed-ridden mother, she maintains a sense of connection with the outside world through her habits of independence, which included home-based employment, her friendships and her acute interest in outside affairs. Like Mr Merton and Mr Allahm, her home embraces the outside world.

Engagement in welfare and community

Another route to outside-connectedness lies in engagement with welfare services and authorities, as suggested by Riley (1988) and Balbo (1991). West German Frau Alexander, who has not worked since before her son's birth, exemplifies this process, as does East German Frau Meissner, who has become employed as a result of her caring career. In both cases, fighting medical and educational officials has generated self-development and confidence in dealing with the public world.

Gaining self-confidence and skills by championing the cause of vulnerable others is a gendered phenomenon. Starting from low clerical positions, neither Frau Alexander nor Frau Meissner has sought to expand her own life opportunities. Yet they threw themselves into fights for their disabled children. As many community and new social movement studies have suggested, the immediacy of the social sphere around women's domestic situations provides a potential springboard to their wider social and political involvement (Campbell, 1996; Mayo, 1994; Miethe, 1999).

While for women welfare issues provide a pathway into the public sphere, for men they provide a route to greater involvement in the private sphere. The new social movements have often been an important vehicle for bringing men into struggles in the sphere of reproduction, which was previously the preserve of women. For social policy, this method of tackling gender inequalities is still in its infancy. Yet Mr Merton, seaman turned caring and disability advocate, provides a striking example of such a switch, triggered by his own experience of disability. The community service alternative to military service in West Germany has provided another route for men into this sphere of politics. Many of the older German women interviewees mentioned their surprise at being tended to in personal tasks by men, and it is known that many Zivis go on to professional training in the medical and social professions. So bringing men into caring may be a highly effective way of breaking down gender divisions and of bolstering the social services system.

Shared cultures

Trust

Networks of the more open kind require a wide level of trust, as Putnam (1993) suggests. The prevalence of informal networking in East Germany was an expression of such widespread trust. We have already commented in chapter three on the high degree of trust in East German work collectives, which seemed surprising in a society permeated by state security surveillance. East German interviewees frequently referred to the loss of trust brought about by unification, by a sudden competition for jobs among workmates, by a fear of who might be outside the door, by new levels of theft and violence. Clearly, such fears reflected the general feeling of insecurity resulting from such a turbulent process of social change, yet it seems that GDR society did generate a strong sense of security. Neighbours happily left their keys with each other and women had no fear of being out alone at night.

Kraemer and Roberts (1996) and Marris (1996) argue that a feeling of ontological security is a prerequisite of outgoing and independent social engagement. Such a sense of security may well be founded in infancy, but is greatly affected by wider social conditions. Wilkinson (1996) associates better health levels with the sense of security attendant on lower levels of inequality and social hierarchy. Social polarisation gives rise to violence and insecurity and higher morbidity levels. This suggests that an important ingredient in East German networking was the level of trust resulting from its relative social homogeneity and low polarisation.

Countercultural energy

We have noted a perverse relationship in each society between the pattern of informal support and what might have been expected from the formal system. East Germany, with the least policy orientation to caring, seemed to engender the strongest web of outer-connectedness. West Germany, whose pluralised system of subsidiarity purports to support the informal sphere of family and community, gave rise to the least socially connected caring situations. In Britain, which advocates individual responsibility, we found a denser mesh of social attachments, although many of them were partial and tentative.

We infer that much of the energy of the informal sphere in East Germany was fuelled by its resistance to the official system. This resistance took the form of overt opposition, but constituted an implicit and commonly shared counterculture, at least among wide sections of the population. (Herr Speyer seemed to exist in a different and smaller counterculture in the private business sector.) Many professionals were sympathetic to carers for resisting official pressure and 'permission' to off-load disabled and elderly members of their families onto poor forms of institutional care. Professionals also officiated for the system, however – hence the tendency of carers to present them as polarised forces of good or evil.

We argued in the chapter on East Germany that the interviewees were giving double testimony, concerning both the old GDR society and their experiences of unification. We noted the way carers tended to intertwine the themes of disability and unification, and interweave their accounts of past and present struggles against bureaucracy, which conveyed a general feeling of being 'up against something'. East Germans in the early 1990s felt that they shared a struggle for survival, which included mastering the new procedures concerning benefits and disability assessments. Knowing that the West German benefits were relatively good, the challenge was to make sure that they got their due, as individuals, as particular occupational groups, and as East Germans. In every housing block there seemed to be individuals who had read all the small print and could help and advise – the informal networks were in full swing!

Britain had experienced a not dissimilar collapse of collectivist principles in welfare, but the carers we interviewed lacked a comparably spirited response. The transition to marketisation and welfare residualism was more attenuated, so the feeling was one of demoralisation rather than outrage. West German benefits were relatively generous, by international as well as East German standards, whereas British benefits had long been and still were in serious decline. And Britain, despite its vigorous voluntary, self-help and community action traditions, seemed to have no generalised infrastructure of networking in place.

There were pockets of resistance in Britain and West Germany. Mr Merton undoubtedly caught his enthusiasm for advocacy work from the disability movement in which his partner was involved. While Mrs Rajan herself made no mention of anti-discrimination movements, her social worker is Asian and her borough is involved in a vigorous process of regeneration in which multiculturalism plays a major part. West Indian Mrs Elliot, who is portrayed in a cameo at the beginning of the book, readily makes and sustains networks, drawing friends in to keep her company at home, where she combines machining with caring. In West Germany, both the Mahlers and the Alexanders are associated with the alternative movement, in the friendship-centredness of their milieus, and in their rather exploitative working of the system of benefits. Frau Alexander and Frau Planck (who is portrayed in cameo at the beginning of the book) rather enjoy their defiance of medical and benefit authorities.

The idea that social energy requires a context of resistance poses a problem for the design of social policy. It is a question long posed by Abrams et al (1989), a pioneer of research into the informal sphere, who has argued that any attempt to organise the informal sphere would spoil its essential spontaneity (Bulmer, 1987). We regard this liberal view, that individual initiative is quelled by organisation, as an over-simplification. The onus is on the welfare system to find ways of supporting spontaneity and creativity; this is the quest of the 'active' approach.

Common social identities

A common social identity which could take many forms seemed integral to the development of supportive relationships between professionals and carers. In the case of Frau Planck, this identification was founded in feminism, and in the Mahlers' case in professionalism. A common class identity seemed to be the critical element in several stories in the West German interviews of visiting physiotherapists or nurses giving carers a diagnosis with which they could challenge the doctor, or identifying a right to a benefit which they could assert against the social assistance office. Such advice never seemed to come from the social assistance office itself, despite the wider social work and medical assessment role of that organisation in the Federal system, and its employment of professionally trained workers. In East Germany, teachers figured prominently, which may be because of their shared abhorrence of poor standards of provision for the most disabled children. As we have said, policies towards disability worked in opposite ways in the two Germanies. In the Federal system, benefits rise in accordance with the severity of the disability; we saw Frau Arndt's legal fight following unification to safeguard her child's assessment as more disabled, in order to maintain a higher benefit level. Under the GDR system, by contrast, parents were anxious to minimise disability, in order to keep their children within the system of education, vocational training and employment. By integrating a disabled child into a mainstream class, teachers could play a critical role in the future of a child and its family.

It may be that universalist principles within education and health give rise to egalitarian attitudes, more so than in the discretionary services. Carter and Everitt (1988), writing of work with older people, contrast the friendship-based and playful style of arts-based adult education with the more hierarchical, even infantilising practices of health promotion and residential care work. They advocate conversation and 'fun' in social practice, and a culture of reciprocity among equals. This culture was achieved by the community worker leading Frau Planck's group, in the supportive relationships between professionals and various carers, and also by a number of carers in groups and networks. Frau Planck's women's group, Frau Arndt's group and the Mahlers' professional network all created a raft of friendship-style support. These are the very relationships which Schwartz (1997) is advocating in seeking to animate a feeling of belonging balanced with a sense of personal autonomy.

Personal support

Partnership

The outwardly oriented carers were much more likely to operate in caring partnerships. Partnership is another aspect of caring which is directly affected by the politics of the sexual division of labour in the home. The Mahlers' and the Grüns' insistence on being interviewed together, and the interweaving of their responses, demonstrated the fullness of their cooperation. Frau Meissner's ex-husband and Frau Alexander's husband were also directly involved in caring tasks. By contrast, the more general West German pattern was for husbands not to be involved in caring as such, but in housebuilding or overtime work. The British husbands were more directly involved in caring, or at least had formerly been when their wives were working (Mr Bally, Mr Buckley). Mr Rajan had tried to help, but Mrs Rajan had rejected his efforts for many years.

Shiftwork promotes the sharing of domestic roles, and full-time employment of couples likewise leads to cooperation. Partnership in caring seems to be associated with networking. We would therefore expect a greater sharing of caring roles among East German couples, as was indeed the case.

In her in-depth study of inter-relationships between conjugal roles and social networks, Bott (1957) found that segregated couple roles were associated with tightly knit networks, and joint roles, in which the couple was a more self-sufficient unit, with loose networks. In our study, loose networking was similarly associated with shared caring roles between partners. As we have seen, an outward orientation can derive from activity in the social sphere as well as from employment. It seems likely that partnership is a precondition of both employment and outside social activity, and that a common capacity to bridge public and private worlds in turn strengthens partner relationships.

Professional support

We have arrived at the question of what kinds of intervention are effective in encouraging participation in informal networks. Schwartz (1997), a follower of Illich[2], argues that the informal sphere flourishes of its own accord, that 'culture' is what people create when left to their own devices, just as grapes ferment. At the same time, his argument for ways of "uncovering and stimulating the submerged impulses of hospitality within the general culture" (p 121) implies that informal cultural life does require intervention, so long as it is of the right kind. Citing the interwar Peckham experiment, which focused on promoting sociability between families as the key to health promotion, he claims that people respond to feeling needed, and that social engagement is often a solution to mental health problems.

The interviews in our study provided several positive examples of professionals launching carers into outside connections through a sustained process of personal support. The network of parents of disabled children to which Frau Arndt belonged had been set up by and continued to meet with the social worker who had initiated it. Frau Arndt clearly liked this person and felt easy with her. The parents and children also met spontaneously as friends, but it seemed that the professional's background role continued to be a mainstay of the group. This group belonged to Lebenshilfe, which ran school and day centres, provided welfare rights, and was vocal in the politics of disability in Leipzig. Thus it was through her relationship with the professional that Frau Arndt's world opened up. The change in Mrs Rajan's caring strategy from home closure to more outside social engagement, training in her child's school, acceptance of respite support and future planning for Bavesh all started from her enjoying the personal support of a social worker. Mrs Buckley's launch into employment was initiated by staff at Great Ormond Street Hospital, who not only gave her moral support but also identified a driving job for her. As long as Melanie continued to have contact with Great Ormond Street over the years, because of her repeated setbacks, Mrs Buckley maintained her pattern of interrupted but full-time employment. Mrs Buckley's liking and respect for the professionals buoyed her up in the face of recurrent problems. They gave her an authoritative model of combining employment with caring.

Frau Planck from West Germany also gained great strength from professional support. By chance she came across a community worker (Sozialpädagogin) who ran a women's group, in which Frau Planck enjoyed social events and bike trips. Participating in the rather outrageous behaviour of a group of women having a good time helped Frau Planck to defy the social prejudice directed at her, at her half-Turkish disabled son and at her low social and educational status. From the group she also gained strength and practical advice for her struggles for discretionary benefits. This seems a good example of Schwartz's argument – Frau Planck's new feeling of belonging fortifies her, and the 'alternative' nature of the group gives piquancy and energy to her previously oppressed and domestically confined existence. The community worker, who is not mentioned in Frau Planck's account beyond their initial encounter, was undoubtedly using group-work techniques.

A quite different form of professional support came to the Mahlers, who were themselves training or qualified in the social work field. Here advice flowed unsolicited in a middle-class professional network of friends. Colleagues thought proactively about the financial advantages of fostering as compared with adoption and about the Mahlers' ambitious plans for communal living with a grandmother and a single-parent friend, and they rang spontaneously with ideas and advice.

Professionals in East Germany sometimes belonged to the same counterculture as the carers who sought their help. Carers' encounters with educational or medical personnel in East Germany were often direct and personal. This was helped by the absence of a bureaucratised system of social security and social services, with personnel locked into a practice of discriminating between deserving and undeserving cases, and of screening clients for eligibility for services and benefits[3]. Particular social provision could of course be abysmal, but the East German carers frequently mentioned particular teachers or doctors who took an interest in their situation and had a liking for the disabled child. This seems more rare among the West German or British cases. The occupational mix in housing estates in East Germany also meant that help might come from a doctor living in the same block, rather than from one in the clinic.

Overall lessons

From this array of social dimensions which support an outward orientation we can firstly conclude that the bridging of public and private worlds is a socially supported achievement, and that an 'ease' in bridging public and private worlds is not lightly attained. Secondly, the spread of relevant dimensions implies many points of entry for social policy interventions, including at the level of wider cultural formations such as patterns of inequality and levels of trust.

Recent policy debates

We now turn to questions of whether community care policies and broader community development approaches in Germany and Britain are in fact oriented to support outward-connectedness. We also consider whether more recent debates concerning the enhancement of social capital or welfare activation seem likely to invigorate informal social cultures. Our argument centres on networking and forms of professional support. Gender changes in employment, despite their significance for caring, are not our focus here.

In West Germany and Britain, there are ongoing debates among professionals and in the wider public domain concerning caring and more general forms of social intervention. The GDR also saw a great many pronouncements, hardly amounting to debate, concerning the 'socialist way of life' and what social arrangements would best further productive participation, including the voluntary effort necessary to bolster the inadequacies of the service sector (Chamberlayne, 1990a, 1992). Given the foreign nature of this discourse to the terms of Western European social policy, in this section we mainly leave it aside, although the informal cultures of East Germany remain an important point of reference.

In comparing policies in Germany and Britain we need to be aware of what needs we are focusing on. If the point of comparison is maintaining caring at a material level, Germany, with its care insurance and rights to respite holidays, is clearly better provided than Britain. Both countries, however, are shifting the delivery of material services to market mechanisms, bringing a culture of accounting and financial management to the fore, which may well undermine the principles of social solidarity on which the voluntary sector has been based (Kaufmann, 1993, p 1000; Hermsen and Weber, 1998, pp 11-12). If social relatedness is a fundamental human need which social policy must be concerned with sustaining and promoting, and if isolation leaves carers 'stuck' and in a situation of considerable crisis, the West German system is failing many carers. If welfare policy should help carers to separate their interests from those of people they care for, make transitions through critical changes in the life course, and achieve empowering forms of personal development and active citizenship, neither system is particularly successful, though there are interesting examples in both societies.

Both societies have been involved in intensive debate concerning home care systems in recent decades. Official concerns have focused on the sometimes inconsistent issues of how to square informal caring with principles of equality and independence for women, and how to deal with the danger of carers themselves becoming ill and financially dependent. In Germany a considerable fanfare surrounded the introduction of care insurance and the development of *Pflegewissenschaft* (care studies) as a new area of vocational training, which would include the community sector *(ambulante Dienste)*. In Britain there has been some discussion of a care insurance scheme, and qualifications in social care are being developed.

Experience of the care insurance scheme in Germany so far indicates that it has had limited impact on the structural conditions of informal caring. A recent study of a West German region found that 87% of older people with care needs were cared for informally, mainly by women and predominantly through kin (partners and children) (Blinkert and Klie, 1999). Evers and colleagues (1997) also estimate that over 80% of applicants for benefits under the care insurance scheme receive informal care through kin and friends (Evers, 1997). In both studies, payments were used to pay carers and/or to pay for individually organised assistance by friends or acquaintances. Thus, payments rather than services are being chosen, although the value of services offered under care insurance is significantly higher. People can also opt for a mixture of services and payments. But Blinkert and Klie found the choice of care mix (informal and formal services) limited to situations in which the informal care arrangements were perceived by applicants as particularly precarious or unstable. Care mix also tended to be used more by male carers (Blinkert and Klie, 1999, p 198; Evers, 1997). It therefore seems that care insurance is stabilising informal care. However, Evers argues that any changes to patterns of informal care resulting from care insurance will take considerable time to filter through, and that local "cultures of care" (sic) will be decisive in determining how care insurance is integrated into particular arenas of community care (1997, p 516).

The number of jobs created as the result of the introduction of the care insurance in Germany has been considerably lower than originally predicted, because the demand for professional care services has not expanded as much as anticipated (Pabst, 1999). Landenberger (1998) regards the marketisation of the care insurance as positive, opening up the community care sector as a space for enhancing professional innovation, learning and competences. But, a lack of demand for professional services will inhibit this potential development unless it is publicly funded. Similarly, in Britain, there is little sign of direct payments for services administered through private agencies enhancing professional skills. And systems of monitoring and review, still in their infancy, are likely to be task- rather than person-oriented.

Both countries have placed emphasis on equality and independence for carers. Yet even carer groups have tended to provide mutual support on practical aspects of caring rather than helping carers to make either personal or social transitions. In our study, instead of propelling carers into wider social connectedness and enhancing social competences, carers groups operated as an extension of the world of caring, further enclosing carers within caring, and substituting other carers or disabled people for prior friends and wider contacts. They helped carers in the important process of coming to terms with caring and disability, but showed few signs of challenging policy, or of addressing the deeper inner forms of pain entailed in caring.

Community care debates in Germany

In Germany, the improvement of basic financing through increased payments for caring (*Pflegegeld*), the automatic right to six weeks of holiday for carers by the systematic provision of residential respite care, the shifting of basic funding of care situations from social assistance to care insurance (*Pflegeversicherung*), and the raising of pension credits to levels equivalent to average earnings, have brought great material improvements and raised the profile of caring. Paradoxically, although these care payments have entailed major national debates, they have forestalled the politicising of carers as a constituency and, despite purporting to redress inequalities between housewives and employed women, have served to mask cuts in other areas (Meyer, 1998). Nor has caring been politicised by feminists in Germany, who have been more concerned with mothers (Chamberlayne, 1997).

Relational work and self-help

While new financial arrangements for caring have clearly not been planned with social relations in mind[4], social relationships have been at the heart of many other debates on social policy in Germany. Relational considerations have been central within mainstream social practice through counselling and education (*Sozialpädagogik*), and in the alternative movement, which achieved a high profile in social policy in the early and mid-1980s, as the Green Party came to national prominence. Both these currents seek to change the bureaucratic hegemony of a complex legal and financial system in which individual benefits are the main point of reference. Common themes include the need for a cultural shift from altruism (*Fremdhilfe*) to self-help as a basis for mobilising the informal sphere, of the need to work with subjective identities and motivations as well as objective conditions, and of the potential within a revamped system of subsidiarity for a fertile interaction between formal and informal resources.

Of course views diverge on these issues. The more cynical view maintains that the informal sphere is being used as a shunting yard for insoluble problems, and that welfare is being reprivatised into the family (Seibel, 1989, p 178). This view argues the need for a 'revolutionary' change in professional practice in order to repair the dislocation between system and life-world. A new facilitation of mutual help among those with shared problems, discretion for street-level workers, partnership and co-production between professionals and non-professionals, and a shift from 'on behalf of' to 'with' and 'by' are advocated by Grunow (1996).

A more positive view considers that substantial changes are being made in the German welfare system, often by welfare clients themselves through social networks, and that existing structures, in which welfare organisations already have one foot in the formal sector and another in the informal, are suited to mobilising self-help and personal engagement (Heinze and Olk, 1984). Plaschke (1984) maintains that subsidiarity creates a state-free terrain, where socio-political actors can work on the social order on the basis of their own social goals. He argues that a social action approach seeks to change basic societal relations, as does feminism, and that the new movements form valuable subcultures. Both approaches build a 'new grammar of life forms', bringing both services and a sense of belonging to excluded groups (*Aussteiger*). Zapf (1986) likewise speaks of a shift in social policy from an emphasis on utility, redistribution and inequality to a focus on satisfaction, belonging and self-realisation (p 142). Keupp (1987) advocates a reorientation towards the need for time, attention and safety.

Some writers argue that carers are continually fobbed off with promises of involvement, with no supporting service commitment, while others maintain that fundamental changes have already taken place. In this view, carers already act as co-decision makers, informal case managers, life planners (in financial affairs) and service brokers. Like Balbo (1991),

Evers (1993) argues that carers' involvement in the social arena acts as a bridge to action and status in the public sphere, that modern household work has become inter-related service work involving management and negotiation, and that this makes explicit the previously hidden relationship between formal and informal spheres.

Women's projects

Social pedagogic thinking supports the widening of social relationships and the breaking down of the family barriers which can be so isolating for women. Already in the 1970s a shift in family policy urged mothers to differentiate their own and others' interests within family life (Munch, 1990). More recently, family centres have been seeking to build new social infrastructures related to the family, associative forms in everyday life, and to "open up a broad field for individual initiative and mutual support" (Hebenstreit-Müller and Pettinger, 1991, p 41). One centre encourages young mothers to build and find networks, and creates a space in which they can experiment with ideas, while another has made "being a carer without giving up on oneself" its leitmotif (p 50). Many women's projects have been initiated by feminists, and Brückner (1995) explores their scope for tackling issues of authority and dependence between professionals and women users. Traditional gender ideologies can remain strong, however, and Hoecklin (1998) reports the extreme difficulty of launching a mothers' centre in rural Bavaria.

Community care debates in Britain

Whereas in Germany the more innovative critiques of the 1980s developed outside the mainstream system, in Britain opposition to the postwar welfare state came from within the government. In Thatcher's Britain, community care served as an emblem both of retrenchment and of the new consumerism in welfare. Much was promised through new forms of planning, partnership, needs assessment, care packages and renewed attempts to heal the rift between health and social services (Baldock, 1994; Lawson and Davies, 1991). Yet assessments were conducted outside established relationships between carers and professionals, fragmentation of functions brought discontinuities in staffing, and professionals became demoralised by regulation and administration (Lewis, 1994; Hadley and Clough, 1996).

Former radical currents were preoccupied in the 1980s and early 1990s with defending postwar welfare principles. Only with the election of New Labour in 1997 did a more fundamental rethinking of pro-welfare positions gather momentum. But in such thinking, debates from North America rather than innovations in European social policy became dominant, resulting in a rift between arguments concerning communitarianism and social capital.

Caring remained politicised in Britain throughout the 1980s and 1990s. There was frequent coverage about carers and caring in the media, a dense national network of carers groups and organisations, and backing from feminist research and writing on caring issues. The enduring feminist focus on caring gave it prominence in social policy teaching. The militancy and effectiveness of the disability lobby, even its disagreements with the caring lobby, assisted in raising the national profile of caring. Nevertheless, despite these strong forces, the gap between the promise of needs assessment and consultative planning and the reality of incorporation and resource reduction inevitably produced a demoralising effect in the politics of care.

Liberalism and the informal sphere

Differences in underlying political philosophies give rise to different understandings of relations between formal and informal systems of welfare in Germany and Britain. While in Germany the concept of subsidiarity embraces both spheres, in the tradition of British liberalism it is important that public and private spheres remain separate. The guarantee of democracy lies in maintaining a division between civil society and the state, but at the same time civil society stops short of the informal social sphere[5]. As Riley (1988) argues, the more the social sphere developed, that "potential earthly heaven, open to perpetual transformability", the more political science retracted its boundaries, to remove its association with women and domesticity (p 49)[6]. Anthropology has always embraced the arena of informal social and political processes just beyond and contiguous with the household, but it has been less closely aligned with social policy than has political science.

There is little British theorisation in social policy of relations between the public and private spheres. An irony of liberalism is that although the private sphere is regarded as the crucible of freedom, it must not be tampered with, and therefore not supported by outside intervention. This 'instinct' has been compounded by the influence of Foucault in British social policy teaching in the 1980s and 1990s, with arguments that intrusion into the private sphere would constitute yet more state control (Foucault, 1977; Knowles, 1999).

Rights and empowerment

Given belief in the incompatibility of public and private arenas, it is perhaps not surprising that much British literature adopts a combative approach to rights, and emphasises individual roles and empowerment (Mayo, 1994). The role of individual 'social entrepreneurs' has figured in more recent writing on urban regeneration (Leadbeater and Goss, 1998). Analysis of relations between professionals and users has also tended to focus on issues of power (Twigg, 1989).

There are many positive aspects to the rights emphasis in British social policy. The diversified system of local government and welfare pluralism create opportunities for experimentation, even in the face of welfare retrenchment, and the politics of difference is well established in vigorous and effective pressure groups, as well as in local government procedures. Disability and minority ethnic politics is much more widespread and influential in Britain than in Germany (Campbell and Oliver, 1997). Empowerment politics incorporates many of the more radical premises of the community action movement in the 1970s, and gives rise to further innovatory ideas (Mayo, 1994). Unfortunately, British carer organisations have tended to move out of this invigorating orbit of the new social movements (Barnes, 1997).

Communitarianism

The ambiguities of New Labour's appeal to communitarianism as the basis of its Third Way are relevant to our concerns with informal cultures of care. Labour's New Deal policies seem to adopt a more personalised approach to welfare and seek to build upon hidden social resources in the informal sphere. They embrace the terminology of social capital, focus on support for parenting and early childhood, and incorporate counselling in the 'welfare to work' programme.

However, there is a tension within these policies between an emancipatory impetus for citizenship, pluralisation and democratisation, and a more conservative moral order of traditional values, duties and responsibilities (Frazer and Lacey, 1993). Gamarnikow and Green (1999), examining the specific field of education action zones, fear that a conservative interpretation of this reform will operate within a traditional normative frame of conventional families, the work ethic and a deficit approach to educational underachievement, all of which will reinforce educational inequalities. An empowerment approach would construct education around community civic engagement and "the critical possibilities of cultural capital", take wider contextual inequalities into account, and treat social networks as the key ingredient of strengthening social capital and combating social exclusion (p 58).

Relational work

As we have already suggested, recent policy developments impact dramatically on the social relations of caring in Britain. Professional discontinuities and demoralisation, the focus on assessments, review and regulation, the ongoing attrition and unpredictability of services, and abrupt shifts in policy and terminology all detract from creating a secure base for vulnerable people and the kind of personalised support which would often be helpful.

Though not often the focus of government policy, attention to relational issues is reviving. Brown and Harris's (1978) study of depression among young mothers, which examined the correlation between self-esteem and social support, is now increasingly referred to. It found intimacy and the existence of a 'confidant' key protective factors against vulnerability to depression (pp 286-7). In their study of mothers with young children, Bell and Ribbens (1994) argue that social networks are essential to identity, emotional independence within marriage and a sense of existential security. Mothers without social links are the most precarious. The trouble is that the professional and service structures adequate for such work have largely been dismantled. Gordon and Donald (1993) argue that embedding community social work services in the social world of human relationships, in attachments to people and in promoting wider social networks, would require a veritable revolution in professional practice (p 167, p 170).

Marris (1996) argues that the disproportionate heaping of uncertainty on certain sections of the population undermines their emotional attachments, compounding their marginalisation. A sense of control and trust leads to a greater taking of chances, both at the individual and at the community level. Comparing disaster situations, he found different emotional capacities of communities in the context of loss to take charge of their situation and maintain a positive, future orientation. Kraemer and Roberts (1996) see a personal sense of security as a precondition for concern for others, arguing that the demise of public services in Britain provokes a pervasive and debilitating sense of anxiety. We have noted the demoralising effect of slow service deterioration on carers in Britain, and the more spirited response of East German carers to the challenges of unification and the sweeping away of familiar collective supports. The longer period of service decline in Britain, the weaker economy, and the absence of countercultural networks seemed key to the difference.

Comparing German and British approaches

The traditions of community organisation are differently grounded in the two societies. In Germany, there is a more embedded discourse concerning the bridging of public and private spheres, with a tension between more conservative and bureaucratised approaches to family and community, and alternative, professional, often feminist approaches which seek to energise self-help, differentiated cultures of belonging and self-development. Interpersonal work receives less emphasis in British community development work, which tends to be oriented to individual rights and the politics of difference and empowerment. The training of social professionals has by now become polarised, with Germany maintaining its emphasis on educational and group-work skills, and Britain increasingly directed towards management and legal work. This creates an uncertainty in the British context as to whether the professional skills any longer exist to carry out the more person-centred work which Third Way policies seem to require. There is a current of thinking in Britain which advocates attention to basic existential securities and the promotion of interdependence, but it is far from reaching government and mainstream training agendas.

Conclusion

Although the carers in our study were only tangentially affected by community development policies, their various difficulties and successes in maintaining outside connections were richly suggestive of the kinds of cultural support required for a more active and subject-centred model of welfare. Our investigations suggest that outward-orientedness among carers is premised upon routes to the outside world, (through employment, participation in networks, or engagement in welfare or community activity), cultural solidarity (through trust, a counterculture or common social identity) and personal support (through partners or professionals). These structural features have much in common with the characteristics of new social movement politics (Hamel, 1995), and indeed the more outwardly oriented carers in West Germany and Britain in our study do tend to be connected with alternative and disability movements.

Barriers for women between home life and wider social engagement had virtually disappeared in East Germany because of structural transformations concerning women's employment, family expectations and facilitative networks. In West Germany and Britain, however, judging by our study, the family all too often still encloses women carers in domestic confinement and isolation, whether through the force of traditional ideologies and family structures, or through the decline of services, which throws carers back on their own private resources. The energy required to maintain outside connections can wear down carers, and the absence or withdrawal of earlier forms of support can return women to a situation of home-centredness. This points to the salience of positive personal and cultural support in caring. In a demoralised context of service withdrawal, Mrs Buckley and Mrs Bally lose their earlier spirited and resourceful responses to the challenges of caring. But with help from social workers, Mrs Rajan is able to emerge from years of crisis and isolation, and Frau Planck is able to defy the conventional prejudices which have blighted her life. Through outer-connectedness, carers add to their biographical resources and become a resource for others – they contribute to social capital.

As our case studies so eloquently demonstrate, what has been courageously gained can be quickly lost. Our comparison of social policy developments in Germany and Britain suggests that, for all the talk of a subject-centred strengthening of the social sphere, nothing like enough is being done in either welfare system to provide and promote the cultural supports necessary to an active model of welfare. Our concluding chapter, pursuing the policy implications of the study, will elaborate some suggestions in this direction.

Notes

[1] Miethe (1999) identifies a similar tension in East Germany, where women regret the loss of their vibrant, kitchen-based, non-institutionalised practice of politics, which was closely aligned with friendships and family life. Since unification, politics has shifted to the formalised public sphere of meeting halls, from which they feel estranged.

[2] The ideas of Illich (1971), an anti-professional libertarian, have been influential in education. He may be seen as a forerunner of the empowerment movement.

[3] Such processes of regulation and selection were removed in a system in which basic income was guaranteed through subsidies for food, clothing, housing, transport and recreation – all the basic requirements of life were integrated into the mainstream economy.

[4] During a feedback visit to Leipzig in 1995, we encountered concern at the unexpected outcomes of the new system of care insurance, such as family members with no experience of or commitment to caring making claims, particularly in the conditions of high unemployment in East Germany.

[5] Somers (1995) traces political sociology's neglect of the terrain of civil society. In arguing the short-sightedness of this, she refers to the democratic revolutions of the 1980s in Eastern Europe, which "appeared to be nourished by a sphere of social life and free associations ... a 'third' space of popular social movements and collective mobilisation, of informal networks and associations, and of community solidarities" (p 230).

[6] By contrast, Comte, the founding father of French sociology, sought to infuse his new social science with 'social feeling' and a 'feminine aspect' which could assist in comprehending human life 'as a whole' (Riley, 1988, p 49).

SEVEN

Conclusion – caring as a political challenge

In their interviews our research subjects reconstructed their past and present understandings of how their caring situation had unfolded and been supported. Our interpretation of their account and their self-presentation, together with contextual knowledge, allowed us to characterise their 'caring strategy', and the 'biographical resources' available to them. In sociological terms, this involved exploring both actions and meanings.

The strategies adopted by carers made a great difference to the scope and prospect of their lives, and to the lives of those they cared for. Mrs Bally and Mrs Buckley, despite their earlier activism, local connections and supportive husbands, both took the decisions concerning their adult children on themselves, and seemed blocked in finding a way forward. Defeated rather than passive by nature, they made few demands on the welfare system, but also contributed little in terms of energetic initiatives or the enhancing of Peter's and Melanie's future prospects. Their demoralisation may well have affected their own health and ability to cope. And, the more they retreated into the private sphere, the less they knew of the outside options and the less confidence they had in outside solutions. Carers who were outwardly-connected brought a wider range of information to biographical work and decision making. They became flexible, energetic and independent agents, able to make long-term plans and manage crises. The Meissners, through their proactive approach and myriad of social contacts, were widely acquainted with opportunities concerning disabled young people, which they avidly pursued. Frau Arndt's circle of friends – parents of disabled children – were similarly connected with *Lebenshilfe's* active role in the city, its new facilities and its rights work. The social sphere of the Meissners and of Frau Arndt was more than an extension and support for the private sphere of caring. it linked them with a wider social world. Outwardly-oriented carers were continually extending their own skills and knowledge, and greatly improving the life chances of their children. They were mobilising and adding to social capital, with two kinds of pay-off. They were extending their own capacities and skills, while their critical demands and ways of operating were also improving and shaping the welfare system.

These patterns pose a double political challenge. First, what can welfare systems offer the demoralised, home-based carer, in whose situation all the most intractable problems of the traditional gender divide are perpetuated? Second, how rapidly can welfare systems learn from, sustain, and promote more widely the dynamic of more outwardly-oriented carers? Our conclusion draws together our reflections on these issues.

Our case studies point to a more differentiated and interactive approach to welfare, which works with biographical, cultural and professional resources. It is an approach which regards social interdependence as the bedrock of autonomy and individual creativity. It is premised on wide social ties, negotiating capacities, and strong and integrated public services about which information is readily available and in which people have trust.

The German sociological concept of *Vergesellschaftung* (socialisation) is helpful here. Vergesellschaftung denotes the interactive process whereby individuals respond to social change through their lives, and social change is brought about through that process. In similar vein, the SOSTRIS project suggested that policy makers and professionals, by seeing individuals as pioneers of social transformation, might find a route to reconnecting social policy with life-worlds (Chamberlayne and Rustin, 1999).

There are signs of a more differentiated, cultural approach to welfare, and new labour market and family forms seem to offer a historic possibility of bridging the longstanding divides between the public, the social and the private. We should remember, however, that attempts to restructure relationships between the individual, the community and the state have often failed. Britain has repeatedly experienced the overriding of self-help movements by centralised bureaucratisation (Green, 1998). The new social movements of the 1970s and 1980s, for example, cut across the public–private divide, providing women and other marginal groups with routes and access to political platforms and identities (Maheu, 1995). Jenson and Phillips (1996) discuss the way third sector power-sharing, open fluidity and advocacy, which seemed to enhance opportunities for civic engagement in the 1970s and 1980s, became shackled through partnership and consultation arrangements, and the marketisation attendant on cuts in public budgets (p 22). We have seen how the alternative movement of the 1980s in West Germany, the 'Spring' initiatives surrounding the overthrow of the GDR regime, and carer groups in

Britain have all succumbed to this process. And, in present-day Germany and Britain, despite a flurry of talk about a more subject-centred approach, administrative and regulatory concerns seem in the ascendancy, pushed on by marketisation and a very abstracted model of individual choice.

One way to avoid a replay of this cycle of disappointment is to define the prerequisites of a cultural approach to welfare more clearly. Our case studies of individuals painfully and creatively piecing together solutions to highly individualised circumstances represent a new trend in welfare research, which has implications for the way welfare is conceived and constructed, and for practice. They demonstrate the need for an approach which intervenes in, understands and negotiates interconnections between, the personal, informal and structural levels.

Our comparative interpretation of case study material contributes to this task of recasting welfare relations and service contexts. In this conclusion we focus on specific policy aspects of a more cultural approach to welfare. We begin with gender issues. We move on to proposals for working with biographical resources and cultural networks and for enhancing professional support, and finish with a comment on the challenge of caring at the European level.

Gender issues

Caring has developed within social policy as a women's issue, its analysis richly impelled by feminism, with relatively little attention to men carers[1]. Our study suggests that gender relations in caring need a much stronger focus. Equal partnering in caring (Mahlers and Grüns) and partner support (Alexanders and Meissners) were crucial ingredients in outward-oriented caring, and two such cases (in Britain) were men. If a key task in social policy is to encourage men to take their full share of responsibility in the domestic sphere, models of men caring, on their own and in partnerships, would be valuable. More in-depth study of situations in which husbands do and do not act as care partners would be helpful to other couples. Mr Rajan's offers of more involvement were rejected by Mrs Rajan for many years; she became more open to his help only as she opened up to the world in general. Herr Hegemann and Herr Blau, both of whom are disabled, and whose wives are struggling with marital role reversal, might be able to be more supportive if they could discuss in more depth the gender issues involved in their relationship.

Whether husbands play a full role in caring may depend on their or their wives' independent choices, or be a function of a practical situation, or of the couple's emotional interaction. These are complex issues, but they are relevant to almost all the cases we have studied. We noted, for example, that Herr Speyer's control over his wife's life in the past feeds his inability to consider residential options now. His exceptional case alerted us to issues of patriarchy in the family of Frau Arndt and in the marriage of Frau Blau, but also to the relative lack of structural support for patriarchy in East German society. This contrasted with the situation in West Germany, where, as in Frau Hamann's case, the patriarchal form of the family business could remain overwhelmingly determinant.

Gender issues are doubly salient in the case of the Buckleys. Mr Buckley's diminishing involvement as a full care partner firstly resides in the gender taboos surrounding his taking his daughter to a public toilet, especially as she reached adolescence, and then concerning her constant bleeding, which the Buckleys felt he could not deal with even at home. Secondly, as Mrs Buckley retreats into home caring, so she becomes more bound up with Melanie, unable to plan her move to independent living, and even, it seems, to discuss such matters on a partnership basis with her husband. In this case, therefore, an intensifying of gender taboos in adolescence combines with service deterioration to produce a reversion to gender-separated caring. This is a chilling example of the retrogressive effects of welfare retrenchment, and of a failure to address gender issues in caring.

Biographical resources

In chapter five we discussed the role of biographical work as central to identity and pathways in modern society, and as the basis of informed and strategic action. We also discussed the understanding of user biographies as essential to a social policy approach which builds on the resources of existing life worlds and encourages moral agency. Chapter Six sought a structural understanding of why so much more biographical work is required in some contexts than in others.

Carers face great personal challenges in confronting medical hierarchies, in accepting disability within the family identity, in making adjustments to changes in power in marriage relationships, in accepting the loss of retirement as leisure, in balancing their own need for outside sociability and identity with the constant demands of caring. We saw the Grüns painfully struggling to find a balance between normalising the disability of their son in order to treat him as an equal, and adjusting to its real extent. We saw Frau Blau battling against her feelings of dependency, but also against the tendency to get revenge for her past subordination by infantilising her husband. We also saw the urgency for him that she resolve these identity questions. Mrs Rushton likewise was tormented by her own violent responses to the relentless needs of her husband. Yet there was little sign of social work intervention in support of the reflexive working through of traumas and life-course transitions.

In general, carers in Britain maintained a greater hold on their own interests and identities and on future developments than did carers in West Germany. This was not due to a greater degree of professional support, but rather to the relative politicising of caring in Britain throughout the 1980s and 1990s, the media coverage and spread of carer organisations, and feminist research and theorising about caring. These elements have played an important role in bringing visibility to carers and have influenced legislation, but have been powerless in the face of the overall deterioration of welfare.

Sociology has highlighted reflexivity as a crucial resource in postmodern society, but in the context of caring in West Germany, much reflexivity was stuck and fruitless. Kulawik (1991-92) argues that in West Germany, "the linkage between the private and the public was probably more visible and therefore accessible to politicisation than in any other Western country" (p 79), which implies that it might be easier for West German than for East German carers to be reflexive about their situation and to move on. Yet West German carers were often in structurally and culturally intractable positions, and lacked the benefits of public discourse concerning caring. Even debates on care insurance in Germany, which followed our fieldwork period, do not seem to have focused on personal aspects of caring, and have not politicised carers as such.

Frau Luchtig's ceaseless and tormented reflexivity could not enable her to stand up to her mother, nor could Frau Hamann's ruminations on her conflicting identities as mother and professional resolve her dilemmas. The weight of their traditional family structures is highlighted by the comparison with East Germany, to which neither situation could have been transposed (except in exceptional situations, as of the private family firm of Herr Speyer). West German carers were walled into their families in a way which had diminished historically in East Germany. While the facilitative, educational approach of Sozialpädagogik sets out to counter the oppressive effects of traditional family ideology, it can have little effect as long as the basic institutional structures remain unchanged. Besides, in our study Sozialpädagogik reached rather few cases.

We have seen that it was carers whose lives lay outside traditional family structures who became outwardly-oriented. Thus the German welfare state faces the task of remedying social incapacities which are of its own making. Balbo (1991, 1997) maintains that modern welfare systems catapult women into modernity. But this study shows that family-centredness (in West Germany) and withdrawal of public services (in Britain) may well impede social engagement and the development of social competence, and that many welfare subjects may need support in developing more active relationships with the public sphere. The point is reinforced by the gender comparison: men's identities automatically span public and private worlds, and husbands tended to advocate outside solutions. It was the absence of gendered barriers between public and private worlds which resulted in East German carers being more able to act in and challenge the public sphere of welfare. In this sense, they were more empowered to start with.

Cultural networks

Informal networks emerged in the interviews as a fortifying resource. Like employment, they create a habit of bridging public and private worlds, acting as a pole of attraction out of the home, widening carers' information base by enlarging their circle of social contacts, and boosting confidence in challenging difficulties and officialdom. Networks based on countercultural opposition, common social identities and trust are far wider in participative scope and more socially productive in their outcomes than is the 'carer involvement' which is implied and practised in care planning in Britain.

Carers were more likely to belong to loose, impersonal, informal networks (Putnam, 1993) where there was a cultural continuity between their everyday life world and the networking. This happened in East Germany in the networking which compensated for service-sector inadequacies in the GDR, and featured in the common struggle for jobs and to master new procedures in the context of unification. In Britain and West Germany, there were also examples of countercultural networking, as in the Alexanders' biker community and Frau Planck's cheeky women's group. These groups boosted these carers' self-esteem and their confidence to challenge officialdom. The Mahlers' professional network was implicitly countercultural in the sense that the radicalism of social professionals in West Germany often emanated from the alternative movement. The disability movement to which Mr Merton had access through his partner was likewise an oppositional new social movement.

The common class or professional identity between the Mahlers and their colleagues brought a particular ease of communication. Their fluid interweaving of public and private resources was remarkable, as was their free and open talking about emotional experiences, which perhaps also flowed from their professional training. The Grüns were also skilled in 'managing while transcending' the public–private divide, in the particular context of the need to protect private life in the dissident movement in East Germany. Generally, the outward-connected carers achieved partnership relations with the formal services, in the manner advocated by newer approaches to social policy. But none of the other carers received such proactive and systematic advice.

Information could flow through self-help groups as well as through sympathetic professionals, especially where relationships were marked by trust and a common social identity. In the 1970s, during Peter Bally's and Melanie Buckley's childhoods, both families seemed involved in networking practices which paralleled the more generalised practice of networking among parents of young children. The balancing of part-time work with childcare in a context of never adequate public services has built up an ingenious patchwork of provision over the years. Perhaps parents of young children, supported by the universal right to education, tend to feel future-oriented, and perhaps the social optimism of the 1960s and 1970s energised demands for services. In both families that sense of social solidarity broke down later on, as their disabled children became adults, and as the services receded. The self-help groups to which they belonged did not seem to weather these transitions. This was perhaps surprising, given the longstanding culture of self-help groups and associational life in Britain. This culture may well have boosted the more idiosyncratic, personally tailored groups set up by Mr Allahm and Mr Merton.

Professional support

The case studies repeatedly showed the significance of professional support in helping carers like Frau Arndt or Mrs Rajan to make transitions, but they also indicated a number of lost opportunities. Professionals could entice carers to step over the domestic wall in a number of ways.

Mrs Rajan's social worker informed her about respite care, making it seem accessible and acceptable, but there was no such mediating advice for Mrs Buckley and Mrs Bally, who needed to be proactively persuaded of the benefits of independent living schemes for young adults. The fact that Mrs Rajan liked her social worker, who was also Asian, made her more open to advice. That Frau Arndt regarded her social worker as a friend clearly bolstered her morale and sociability, which led on to further developments for herself and for her son. The quality and continuity of these relationships were crucial. Regular home visits from a psychologist or physiotherapist in West Germany built up trust, leading carers to act on such workers' apparently chance remarks concerning a diagnosis or benefit.

We have argued in chapter five that the timing of professional interventions would be helped by a biographical understanding of how transitions and changes relate to earlier experiences. Understanding the generic nature of effective help, which often might not be specifically to do with caring, could greatly expand the opportunities for intervening, even with the most 'stuck' cases like Frau Hegemann or Frau Jakob. Frau Planck's women's group was not concerned with caring. Our case studies showed that realising and expressing anger at their exploited and unrecognised position could raise energy levels and drive carers on a path of tackling authorities and expanding their social competence. Helping carers to build positively on their frustration could therefore be one form of intervention. Helping them to tackle the personal and hidden traumas of caring, or to break an internalised gender barrier by accepting and encouraging help from a partner would be very different exercises. Carers often need diverse and imaginative professional work, backed by in-depth training in counselling and community work skills, along the lines of Sozialpädagogik.

An individualised approach might be thought to lead to the conclusion that since many carers find their own ways to mobilise resources and support, interventions by professionals are not needed. That would neglect the painful and slow process by which many carers have reached their solutions, and the situations of carers who are stuck. It would also neglect the opportunity of using the more active carers as models for other carers, and as models of active welfare subjects in new thinking about social policy in general. It would also deny the main message of our findings, that an outward orientation needs to be structurally supported by services and networks, and personally supported by partners and professionals. This is especially the case in societies in which traditional family forms and ideologies remain in place.

Implications at the European level

In recent years, European concern with gender issues has extended towards the goal of equality between the productive and reproductive spheres. Leave for family reasons, pension credits and payments for caring are receiving attention. Our study suggests that the social sphere is also critically important in the democratisation of welfare, by combining support for home caring with pathways to civic engagement and personal development. This requires a new integration of gender, life-world and third-sector research.

European comparative research creates opportunities for fresh thinking about social policy, sharing best practice and piecing together the strengths of each system. Imagine a combination of all the worst facets: the sense of insecurity and abandonment from the demise of services, as in Britain; isolated confinement in family structures and ideologies, as in West Germany; appalling standards of residential services and callous medical attitudes, as in the GDR. By contrast, the best of all possible worlds includes: a culture of energetic and resourceful (and quite likely oppositional) informal networks, as in the GDR and in the new social movements in West Germany and Britain; a reliable infrastructure of robust and properly coordinated services; supportive and personalised relations with professionals who are skilled in holistic and community work. From this there would be extraordinary benefits in terms of generating social competence and social capital, gender equality, lifelong learning, social trust and management of change and transitions.

Notes

[1] There has been some attention in research to men carers: for example, the high incidence of older men caring for their disabled wives, the effects on marital relations of caring between spouses, the higher level of services offered to men carers, and men's different definition of and approach to caring (for example Arber and Gilbert, 1989; Parker, 1990).

Bibliography

Abrams, P., Abrams, S., Humphrey, R. and Snaith, R. (1989) *Neighbourhood care and social policy*, London: HMSO.

Ackers, L. (1999) *Shifting spaces: Women, citizenship and migration within the European Union*, Bristol: The Policy Press.

Adams, P. (1990) 'The unity of economic and social policy in the German Democratic Republic', in B. Deacon and J. Szalai (eds) *Social policy in the new Eastern Europe*, Aldershot: Avebury.

Ahmad, W.I.U. and Atkin, K. (eds) (1996) *'Race' and community care*, Buckingham: Open University Press.

Althammer, J. and Pfaff, A.B. (1999) 'Materielle und soziale Sicherung von Frauen in der Perspektive des Lebenslaufs', *Monatszeitschrift des Wirtschafts- und Sozialwissenschaftlichen Instituts in der Heinz-Böckler-Stiftung (WSI-Mitteilungen)*, pp 32-40.

Anderson, P. (1999) 'The German question', *London Review of Books*, 7 January 1999, pp 10-16.

Angerhausen, S., Backhaus-Maul, H. and Schiebel, M. (1993) *In 'guter Gemeinschaft'? Die sozial-kulturelle Verankerung von intermediären Organisationen im Sozialbereich der neuen Bundesländer*, ZfS-Arbeitspapier 14, Bremen: Zentrum für Sozialpolitik, University of Bremen.

Apitzsch, U. and Inowlocki, L. (2000) 'Biographical analysis: a German school?', in P. Chamberlayne, J. Bornat and T. Wengraf (eds) *The turn to biographical methods in social science: Comparative issues and examples*, London: Routledge.

Atkin, K. (1991) 'Health, illness, disability and black minorities: a speculative critique of present-day discourse', *Disability, Handicap and Society*, vol 6, no 1, pp 37-47.

Backhaus-Maul, H. and Olk, T. (1993) 'Von der staatssozialistischen zur kommunalen Sozialpolitik; Gestaltungsspielräume und -probleme bei der Entwicklung der Sozial-, Alten- und Jugendhilfe in den neuen Bundesländern', *Archiv für Kommunalwissenschaften*, vol 2, pp 301-30.

Balbo, L. (1987) 'Family, women and the state: notes towards a typology of family roles and public intervention', in C.S. Maier (ed) *Changing boundaries of the political*, Cambridge: Cambridge University Press.

Balbo, L. (1991) 'Crazy quilts: rethinking the welfare state debate from a woman's point of view', in A. Showstack Sassoon (ed) *Women and the state*, London: Hutchinson.

Baldock, J. (1994) 'The personal social services: the politics of care', in V. George and S. Miller (eds) *Social policy towards 2000*, London: Routledge.

Baldock, J. (1998) 'Old age, consumerism and the social care market', in E. Brunsdon, H. Dean and R. Woods (eds) *Social Policy Review 10*, pp 165-82, London: Social Policy Association.

Baldock, J. (1999) 'Social services and contrary cultures', in P. Chamberlayne, A. Cooper, R. Freeman and M. Rustin (eds) *Welfare and culture in Europe: Towards a new paradigm in social policy,* London: Jessica Kingsley.

Baldock, J. and Ungerson, C. (1994) *Becoming consumers of community care: Households within the mixed economy of welfare*, Community Care into Practice Series, York: Joseph Rowntree Foundation.

Banks, S. (1995) *Ethics and values in social work*, Basingstoke: Macmillan.

Barnes, C., Mercer, G. and Shakespeare, T. (1999) *Exploring disability: A sociological introduction,* Cambridge: Polity Press.

Barnes, H. (1997) *Care, communities and citizens*, London: Longman.

Barnes, M. and Walker, A. (1996) 'Consumerism versus empowerment: a principled approach to the involvement of older service users', *Policy & Politics,* vol 24, no 4, pp 375-93.

Bauer, R. (1985) 'Die Politik der "freien Träger": Aufgabenfelder, Handlungsorientierungen und Leistungspotentiale', in J. Krüger and E. Pankoke, (eds) *Kommunale Sozialpolitik*, Munich: Oldenbourg.

Beck, U. (1992) *Risk society: Towards a new modernity*, London: Sage Publications.

Becker, U. (1989) 'Frauenerwerbstätigkeit – eine vergleichende Bestandsaufnahme', in *Aus Politik und Zeitgeschichte*, Supplement to *Das Parlament*, vol 28/29, 7 July, pp 22-33.

Bell, L. and Ribbens, J. (1994) 'Isolated houswives and complex maternal worlds: the significance of social contacts between women and young children in industrial societies', *The Sociological Review*, vol 42, pp 227-62.

Bennington, J. and Taylor, M. (1993) 'Changes and challenges facing the UK welfare state in Europe in the 1990s', *Policy & Politics*, vol 21, no 2, pp 121-34.

Berger, P. and Luckmann, T. (1967) *The social construction of reality: A treatise in the sociology of knowledge*, Harmondsworth: Penguin.

BerlinOnLine (2000) *Finanzkrise der Pflegeversicherung grösser als angenommen*, BerlinOnline GmbH, 12 August.

Bertram, H. (1992) *Die Familie in den neuen Bundesländern: Stabilität und Wandel in der gesellschaftlichen Umbruchsituation*, Opladen: Leske und Budrich.

Blinkert, B. and Klie, T. (1999) *Pflege im sozialen Wandel: Eine Untersuchung zur Situation häuslich versorgter Pflegebedürftiger nach Einführung der Pflegeversicherung*, Hannover: Vincentz Verlag.

Bochel, C. and Bochel, H. (1998) 'The governance of social policy', in E. Brunsdon, H. Dean and R. Woods (eds) *Social Policy Review*, no 10, pp 57-74, London: Social Policy Association.

Böckmann-Schewe, L., Kulke, C. and Röhrig, A. (1995) '"Es war immer so, den goldenen Mittelweg zu finden zwischen Familie und Beruf war eigentlich das Entscheidende." Kontinuitäten und Veränderungen im Leben von Frauen in den Neuen Bundesländern', *Berliner Journal für Soziologie*, vol 2, pp 207-22.

Born, C. and Krüger, H. (1993) *Erwerbsverläufe von Ehepartnern und die Modernisierung weiblicher Lebensläufe*, Berlin: Deutscher Studienverlag.

Bott, E. (1957) *Family and social network: Roles, norms, and external relationships in ordinary urban families*, London: Tavistock.

Bradley Scharf, C. (1984) *Politics and change in East Germany: An evaluation of socialist democracy*, London: Pinter.

Braye, M. and Preston-Shoot, M. (1995) *Empowering practice in social care*, Buckingham: Open University Press.

Breckner, R. (1997) 'The biographical-interpretive method – principles and procedures', in *SOSTRIS working paper 2: Case study materials on the early retired*, London: University of East London, Centre for Biography in Social Policy, pp 91-104.

Breckner, R., Hungerbühler, W. and Olk, T. (1999) 'An agency in times of transition: the "Bauhof" in Halle', in *SOSTRIS working paper 8: Innovative social agencies in Europe*, London: University of East London, Centre for Biography in Social Policy, pp 65-74.

Brown, G. and Harris, T. O. (1978) *The social origins of depression*, London: Tavistock.

Brückner, M. (1995) 'Professional feminists caught between solidarity and disappointment: the German case', *The European Journal of Women's Studies*, vol 2, pp 77-94.

Bulmer, M. (1987) 'Privacy and confidentiality as obstacles to interweaving formal and informal social care: the boundaries of the private realm', *Journal of Voluntary Action Research*, vol 16, pp 11-25.

Bury, M. (1982) 'Chronic illness: a biographical disruption', *Sociology of Health and Illness*, vol 14, no 2, pp 167-82.

Campbell, B. (1996) 'Gender crisis and community', in S. Kraemer and J. Roberts (eds) *The politics of attachment: Towards a secure society*, London: Free Association Books.

Campbell, J. and Oliver, M. (1997) *Disability politics: Understanding our past, changing the future*, London: Routledge.

Carter, P. and Everitt, A. (1988) 'Conceptualising practice with older people: friendship and conversation', *Ageing and Society*, vol 18, pp 79-99.

Chamberlayne, P (1990a) 'Neighbourhood and tenant participation in the GDR', in B. Deacon and J. Szalai (eds) *Social policy in the new Eastern Europe*, Aldershot: Avebury.

Chamberlayne, P. (1990b) 'The mothers' manifesto and the debate over Mütterlichkeit', *Feminist Review*, no 35, pp 9-23.

Chamberlayne, P. (1993) 'Models of welfare and informal care', in J. Twigg (ed) *Informal care in Europe*, York: University of York, Social Policy Research Unit.

Chamberlayne, P. (1994) 'Women and social policy in Germany', in J. Clasen and M. Freeman (eds) *Social policy in Germany*, Hemel Hempstead: Harvester Wheatsheaf.

Chamberlayne, P. (1995) 'Self-organisation and older people in Eastern Germany', in G. Craig and M. Mayo (eds) *Community empowerment: A reader in participation and development*, London: Zed Books.

Chamberlayne, P. (1997) 'Fürsorge und Pflege in der britischen feministischen Diskussion', *Feministische Studien*, vol 14, no 2, pp 47-60.

Chamberlayne, P. (1999) Beyond the wall: changing political cultures of the informal sphere, *Soundings*, issue 11 on emotional labour, pp 167-75.

Chamberlayne, P. and King, A. (1996) 'Biographical approaches in comparative work: the Cultures of Care project', in L. Hantrais and S. Mangen (eds) *Cross-national research methods in the social sciences*, London: Pinter.

Chamberlayne, P. and Rustin, M. (1999) *From biography to social policy: final report of the SOSTRIS project*, SOSTRIS Working Paper 9, London: University of East London, Centre for Biography in Social Policy.

Chamberlayne, P., Bornat, J. and Wengraf, T. (eds) (2000) *The turn to biographical methods in social science: Comparative issues and examples*, London: Routledge.

Chamberlayne, P., Cooper, A., Freeman R. and Rustin, M. (eds) (1999) *Welfare and culture in Europe: Towards a new paradigm in social policy*, London: Jessica Kingsley.

Clarke, J. (1996) 'After social work?', in N. Parton (ed) *Social theory, social change and social work*, London: Routledge.

Clasen, J. and Freeman, R. (1994) 'The German social state: an introduction', in J. Clasen and M. Freeman (eds) *Social policy in Germany*, Hemel Hempstead: Harvester Wheatsheaf.

Cooper, A. (1999) 'Introduction to part II', in P. Chamberlayne, A. Cooper, R. Freeman and M. Rustin (eds) *Welfare and culture in Europe: Towards a new paradigm in social policy*, London: Jessica Kingsley.

Cooper, A. (2000) 'The vanishing point of resemblance: comparative welfare as philosophical anthropology', in P. Chamberlayne, J. Bornat and T. Wengraf (eds) *The turn to biographical methods in social science: comparative issues and examples*, London: Routledge.

Corbin, J. M. and Strauss, A. (1988) *Unending work and care: Managing chronic illness at home*, San Francisco: Jossey Bass.

Deakin, N. (1994) *The politics of welfare*, Hemel Hempstead: Harvester Wheatsheaf.

Department of Health (1996) *Personal social services: Local authority statistics*, London: HMSO.

Department of Health (1997) *Community care statistics 1997: residential personal social services for adults, England*, London: HSMO.

Department of Health (1998) *Modernising health and social services. National priorities guidelines 1999/00-2001/02*, London: Department of Health.

Dölling, I. (1994) 'Women's experiences "above" and "below": how East German women experience and interpret their situation after the unification of the two German states', *The European Journal of Women's Studies*, vol 1, pp 29-42.

Dölling, I. (1995) 'Zum Verhältnis von modernen und traditionalen Aspekten im Lebenszusammenhang von Frauen in der DDR', in Zentrum für interdisziplinäre Frauenforschung der Humboldt-Universität Berlin (ed) *Unter Hammer und Zirkel: Frauenbiographien vor dem Hintergrund ostdeutscher Sozialisationserfahrungen*, Pfaffenweiler: Centaurus.

Domingues, J. M. (2000) 'Social integration, system integration and collective subjectivity', *Sociology*, vol 34, no 2, pp 225-41.

Donati, P. (1995) 'Identity and solidarity in the complex of citizenship: the relational approach', *International Sociology*, vol 10, no 3, pp 299-314.

Douglas, A. and Philpott, T. (1998) *Caring and coping*, London: Routledge.

Duncombe, J. and Marsden, D. (1993) 'Love and intimacy: the gender division of emotion and "emotion work"', *Sociology*, vol 27, pp 221-41.

Elias, N. (1980) *Über den Prozess der Zivilisation* (2 vols), Frankfurt a.M.: Suhrkamp.

Emery, F.E. (1969) *Systems thinking: Selected readings*, Harmondsworth: Penguin.

Esping-Andersen, G. (1990) *The three worlds of welfare capitalism*, London: Polity.

Evers, A. (1993) 'Diversity and transition: the interaction of professional and informal helpers in home-based care services for elderly people', in J. Twigg (ed) *Informal care in Europe,* York: University of York, Social Policy Research Unit.

Evers, A. (1997) 'Geld oder Dienste? Zur Wahl und Verwendung von Geldleistungen im Rahmen der Pflegeversicherung', *Monatszeitschrift des Wirtschafts- und Sozialwissenschaftlichen Instituts in der Heinz-Böckler-Stiftung (WSI-Mitteilungen),* no 7, pp 510-18.

Evers, A. and Rauch, U. (1999) 'Ambulante Altenpflege – Umbau oder Abbau kommunaler Verantwortlichkeit', *Zeitschrift für Sozialreform,* vol 45, no 2, pp 170-85.

Ferree, M. (1993) 'The rise and fall of "mommy politics": feminism and unification in (East) Germany', *Feminist Studies,* vol 19, no 1, pp 89-115.

Finch, J. (1989) *Family obligation and social change,* Cambridge: Polity.

Finch, J. and Groves, D. (1983) *A labour of love: Women, work and caring,* London: Routledge and Kegan Paul.

Finch, J. and Mason, J. (1993) *Negotiating family responsibilities,* London: Routledge.

Fischer-Rosenthal, W. (2000) 'Biographical work and biographical structuring in present-day societies', in P. Chamberlayne, J. Bornat and T. Wengraf (eds) *The turn to biographical methods in social sciences: Comparative issues and examples,* London: Routledge.

Focus Consultancy Ltd (1993) *Caring for people who live at home: A Focus research report into the community care needs of Newham's black and ethnic minority communities,* London: Newham Social Services Department.

Foucault, M. (1977) *Discipline and punish: The birth of the prison,* (translated by A. Sheridan), London: Penguin.

Frazer, E. and Lacey, N. (1993) *The politics of community: A feminist critique of the liberal-communitarian debate,* Hemel Hempstead: Harvester Wheatsheaf.

Freeman, R. and Rustin, M. (1999) 'Introduction: welfare, culture and Europe', in P. Chamberlayne, A. Cooper, R. Freeman and M. Rustin (eds) *Welfare and culture in Europe: Towards a new paradigm in social policy*, London: Jessica Kingsley.

Frevert, U. (1984*)*, *Krankheit als politisches Problem 1770-1880*, Göttingen: Vandenhoek und Ruprecht.

Gamarnikow, E. and Green, A. (1999) 'Developing social capital: dilemmas, possibilities and limitations in education', in A. Hayton (ed) *Tackling disaffection and social exclusion*, London: Kogan Page.

Geertz, C. (1975) *The interpretation of cultures*, London: Hutchinson.

Gerhard, U. (1991-92) 'German women and the costs of unification', *German Politics and Society*, nos 24-5, pp 16-33.

Giddens, A. (1991) *Modernity and self-identity: Self and society in the late modern age*, Cambridge: Polity.

Glaser, B. and Strauss, A. (1967) *The discovery of grounded theory: Strategies for qualitative research*, New York: Aldine de Gruyter.

Glendinning, C. and Bewley, C. (1992) *Involving disabled people in community care planning: The first steps*, Manchester: University of Manchester, Department of Social Policy and Social Work, University of Manchester Press.

Gordon, D. S. and Donald, S. C. (1993) *Community social work, older people and informal care: A romantic illusion?*, Aldershot: Avebury.

Gottfried, H. (1998) 'Beyond patriarchy? Theorising gender and class', in *Sociology*, vol 32, no 3, pp 451-68.

Graham, H. (1983) 'The social context of caring', in J. Finch and D. Groves (eds) *A labour of love: Women, work and caring*, London: Routledge and Kegan Paul.

Graham, H. (1991) 'The concept of caring in feminist research: the case of domestic service', *Sociology*, vol 25, no 1, pp 61-78.

Green, D. (1998) 'Mutuality and voluntarism: a "third way" for welfare reform?' *Social Policy Review*, no 10, pp 75-84.

Grunow, D. (1996) 'Debureaucratisation and the self-help movement: towards a restructuring of the welfare state in the Federal Republic of Germany', in R. Hadley and R. Clough (eds) *Care in chaos: Frustration and challenge in community care*, London: Cassell.

Hadley, R. and Clough, R. (1996) *Care in chaos: Frustration and challenge in community care*, London: Cassell.

Haley, J. (1963) *Strategies of psychotherapy*, New York: Grune and Stratton.

Hamel, P. (1995) 'Collective action and the paradigm of individualism', in L. Maheu (ed) *Social movements and social classes: The future of collective action*, London: Sage Publications.

Hann, C. and Dunn, E. (1996) *Civil society: Changing western models,* London: Routledge.

Hartley, D. (1994) 'Social security', in V. George and S. Miller (eds) *Social policy towards 2000: Squaring the welfare circle*, London: Routledge.

Hebenstreit-Müller, S. and Pettinger, R. (eds) (1991) *Miteinander lernen, leben, engagieren – neue soziale Netze für familien*, Bielefeld: Kleine Verlag.

Heinze, R. and Olk, T. (1984) 'Rückzug des Staates: Aufwertung der Wohlfahrtsverbände?', in R. Bauer and H. Diessenbacher, (eds) *Organisierte Nächstenliebe: Wohlfahrtsverbände und Selbsthilfe in der Krise des Sozialstaats*, Opladen: Westdeutscher Verlag.

Hermsen, T. and Weber, M. (1998) 'Die freie Wohlfahrtspflege im Spannungsfeld einer Sozialpolitik zweiter Ordnung und neuer Steuerungsmodelle in Kommunen', *Arbeit und Sozialpolitik*, nos 11-12, pp 61-8.

Hervey, T. and Shaw, J. (1998) 'Women, work, and care: women's dual role and double burden in EC sex equality law', *Journal of European Social Policy*, vol 8, no 1, pp 43-63.

Hildebrandt, R. (1994) 'Die Einrichtungen des Gesundheits- und Sozialwesens in der DDR und in den neuen Bundesländern', *Aus Politik und Zeitgeschichte,* vol 3, pp 15-25.

Hirst, P. (1994) *Associative democracy*, Cambridge: Polity Press.

Hochschild, A. (1979) 'Emotion work, feeling rules, and social structure', *American Journal of Sociology*, vol 85, no 3, pp 551-75.

Hochschild, A. (1989) *The second shift: Working parents and the revolution at home*, London: Judy Piatkus.

Hoecklin, L. (1998) '"Equal but different": welfare, gender ideology and a "mother's centre" in southern Germany', in I. R. Edgar and A. Russell (eds) *The anthropology of welfare*, London: Routledge.

Hofmann, M. (1991) *Aufbruch im Warteland: Ostdeutsche soziale Bewegungen im Wandel*, Bamberg: Palette Verlag.

Holstein, J. and Gubrium J. (1994) 'Constructing family: descriptive practice and domestic order', in T. R. Sarbin and J. I. Kitsuse (eds) *Constructing the social*, New York: Sage.

Holzhausen, E. (1997) *Still battling? The Carers' Act one year on*, London: Carers National Association.

Hoyes, L. and Means, R. (1993) 'Quasi-markets and the reform of community care', in J. Le Grand and W. Bartlett (eds) *Quasi-markets and social policy*, London: Macmillan.

Hoyes, L., Jeffers, S., Lart, R., Means, R. and Taylor, M. (1993) *User empowerment and the reform of community care: An interim assessment*, Bristol: University of Bristol, School for Advanced Urban Studies.

Illich, I. (1971) *Deschooling society*, New York, NY: Harper and Row.

Jarausch, K. (1998) 'Realer Sozialismus als Fürsorgediktatur: zur begrifflichen Einordnung der DDR', *Aus Politik und Zeitgeschichte*, B20, pp 33-46.

Jenson, J. and Phillips, S. (1996) *Citizenship regimes: From equity to marketisation*, Florence: European University Institute.

Jones, C. and Rupp, S. (2000) 'Understanding the carers' world: a biographic interpretive case study', in P. Chamberlayne, J. Bornat and T. Wengraf (eds) *The turn to biographical methods in social science: Comparative issues and examples*, London: Routledge.

Joseph Rowntree Foundation (1996) *Meeting the cost of care*, York: Joseph Rowntree Foundation.

Kaufmann, F.X. (1993) 'Artikel Sozialpolitik', in G. Enderle (ed) *Lexikon der Wirtschaftsethik*, pp 998-1005, Freiburg: Herder.

Keady, J. and Nolan, M. R. (1994) 'Younger onset dementia: developing a longitudinal model as the basis for a research agenda and as a guide to interventions with sufferers and carers', *Journal of Advanced Nursing*, vol 19, no 4, pp 659-69.

Kemmer, D. (2000) 'Tradition and change in domestic roles and food preparation', *Sociology*, vol 34, no 2, pp 323-33.

Kendall, J. and Knapp, M. (1997) 'The United Kingdom', in L. M. Salamon and H. K. Anheier (eds) *Defining the non-profit sector: A cross-national analysis*, Manchester: Manchester University Press.

Kesselheim, H. (1999) 'Pflegeversicherung – quo vadis?', *Arbeit und Sozialpolitik*, nos 3-4, pp 57-61.

Keupp, H. (1987) 'Soziale Netzwerke – eine Metapher des gesellschaftlichen Umbruchs?', in H. Keupp and B. Röhrle (eds) *Soziale Netzwerke*, Frankfurt/Main: Campus.

King, A. (2000) 'Part of the system: the experience of home-based caring in West Germany', in P. Chamberlayne, J. Bornat and T. Wengraf (eds) *The turn to biographical methods in social science: Comparative issues and examples*, London: Routledge.

King, A. and Chamberlayne, P. (1996) 'Comparing the informal sphere: public and private relations of welfare in East and West Germany', *Sociology*, vol 30, no 4, pp 741-61.

Klett-Davies, M. (1997) 'Single mothers in Germany: supported mothers who work', in S. Duncan and R. Edwards (eds) *Single mothers in an international context: Mothers or workers?*, London: University of London Press.

Knijn, T. and Kremer, M. (1997) 'Gender and the caring dimension of welfare states: towards inclusive citizenship', *Social Politics*, vol 4, no 3, pp 328-61.

Knowles, C. (1999) 'Cultural perspectives and welfare regimes: the contributions of Foucault and Lefebvre', in P. Chamberlayne, A. Cooper, R. Freeman and M. Rustin (eds) *Welfare and culture in Europe: Towards a new paradigm in social policy*, London: Jessica Kingsley.

Kofman, E. and Sales, R. (1996) 'The geography of gender and welfare in Europe', in M.D. Garcia-Ramon and J. Monks (eds) *Women of the European Union: The politics of work and daily life*, London: Routledge.

Kraemer, S. and Roberts, J. (eds) (1996) *The politics of attachment: Towards a secure society*, London: Free Association Books.

Krisch, H. (1985) *The GDR: The search for identity*, Boulder: Colorado Press.

Kulawik, T. (1991-92) 'Autonomous mothers? West German feminism reconsidered', *German Politics and Society*, nos 24-5, pp 67-85.

Landenberger, M. (1998) *Innovatoren des Gesundheitssystems*, Bern: Huber.

Langan, M. and Ostner, I. (1991) 'Gender and welfare', in G. Room (ed) *Towards a European welfare state?*, Bristol: University of Bristol, School for Advanced Urban Studies.

Lawson, R. and Davies, B. (1991) 'The home-help service in England and Wales', in A. Jamieson (ed) *Home care for older people in Europe: A comparison of policies and practice*, Milton Keynes: Open University Press.

Layder, D. (1998) *Sociological practice: Linking theory and social research,* London: Sage Publications.

Leadbeater, C. and Goss, S. (1998) *Civic entrepreneurship*, London: Demos.

Le Grand, J. and Bartlett, W. (1993) 'Introduction', in J. Le Grand and W. Bartlett (eds) *Quasi-markets and social policy*, London: Macmillan.

Leibfried, S. (1993) 'Towards a European welfare state?', in C. Jones (ed) *New perspectives on the welfare state in Europe*, London: Routledge.

Leibfried, S. and Ostner, I. (1991) 'The particularism of West German welfare capitalism', in M. Adler, C. Bell and A. Sinfield (eds) *The sociology of social security*, Edinburgh: Edinburgh University Press.

Leibfried, S. and Tennstedt, F. (1985) 'Einleitung', in S. Leibfried and F. Tennstedt (eds) *Politik der Armut und die Spaltung des Sozialstaats,* Frankfurt: Suhrkamp.

Leisering, L. and Leibfried, S. (1999) *Time and poverty in Western welfare states. United Germany in perspective,* Cambridge: Cambridge University Press.

Lewis, J. (1992) 'Gender and the development of welfare regimes', *Journal of European Social Policy*, vol 2, no 3, pp 159-73.

Lewis, J. (1993) 'Introduction: women, work, family and social policies in Europe', in J. Lewis (ed.) *Women and social policies in Europe. Work, family and the state*, Aldershot: Edward Elgar.

Lewis, J. (1994) 'Choice, needs and enabling: the new community care', in A. Oakley and A.S. Williams (eds) *The Politics of the welfare state*, London: UCL Press.

Lewis, J. and Glennerster, H. (1998) *Implementing the new community care,* Buckingham: Open University Press.

Lewis, J. and Meredith, B. (1988) *Daughters who care: Daughters caring for mothers at home*, London: Routledge.

Lewis, J. and Ostner, I. (1992) *Gender and the evolution of European social policy,* Working Paper No 7/92, Bremen: University of Bremen, Centre for Social Policy Research.

Lorenz, W. (1994) 'Personal social services', in J. Clasen and M. Freeman (eds) *Social policy in Germany*, Hemel Hempstead: Harvester Wheatsheaf.

Madeley, J. (1991) 'Politics and religion in Western Europe', in G. Moyser (ed) *Politics and religion in the modern world*, London: Routledge.

Mädje, E. and Neusüss, C. (1994) 'Lone mothers on welfare in West Berlin: disadvantaged citizens or women avoiding patriarchy?', *Environment and Planning A*, vol 26, pp 1419-33.

Maier, C. (1997) *Dissolution: The crisis of communism and the end of East Germany*, Princeton, NJ: Princeton University Press.

Marris, P. (1996) *The politics of uncertainty: Attachment in private and public life*, London: Routledge.

Mayo, M. (1994) *Communities and caring: The mixed economy of welfare*, London: St Martin's.

Means, R. and Smith, R. (1994) *Community care policy and practice,* London: Macmillan.

Merkel, I. (1994) 'Leitbilder und Lebensweisen von Frauen in der DDR', in H. Kälble, J. Kocke and H. Zwar (eds) *Sozialgeschichte der DDR*, Stuttgart: Klett-Cotta.

Meyer, T. (1998) 'Retrenchment, reproduction, modernisation: pension politics and the decline of the German breadwinner model', *Journal of Social Policy*, vol 8, no 3, pp 195-211.

Michalsky, H. (1984) 'Social policy and the transformation of society', in K. von Beyme and H. Zimmermann (eds) *Policy making in the German Democratic Republic*, New York: St Martin's Press.

Miethe, I. (1999) 'From "mother of the revolution" to "fathers of unification": concepts of politics among women activists following unification', *Social Politics*, vol 6, no 1, pp 1-22.

Moller Okin, S. (1991) *Justice, gender and the family*, New York, NY: Basic Books.

Morris, J. (1993) *Independent lives: Community care and disabled people*, Basingstoke: Macmillan.

Munch, U. (1990) *Familienpolitik in der Bundesrepublik Deutschland: Massnahmen, Defizite, Organisation familienpolitischer Staatstätigkeit*, Freiburg: Lambertus.

Nolan, M. and Grant, G. (1993) 'Rust out and therapeutic reciprocity: concepts to advance the nursing care of older people', *Journal of Advanced Nursing*, vol 18, pp 1305-14.

Nolan, M., Grant, G. and Keady, J. (1996) *Understanding family care*, Buckingham: Open University Press.

Oakley, A. and Williams, A. S. (eds) *The politics of the welfare state*, London: UCL Press.

Offe, C. (1991) 'Die deutsche Vereinigung als "natürliches Experiment"', in B. Giesen and C. Leggewie (eds) *Experiment Vereinigung: Ein sozialer Grossversuch*, Berlin: Rotbuch.

Oliver, M. (1994) 'Moving on: from welfare paternalism to welfare citizenship', *Journal of the Centre for Social Action*, vol 2, no 1.

Olk, T. (1986) 'Neue Subsidiaritätspolitik – Abschied vom Sozialstaat oder Entfaltung autonomer Lebensstile?', in R.G. Heinze (ed) *Neue Subsidiarität: Leitidee für eine zukünftige Sozialpolitik?*, Opladen: Westdeutscher Verlag.

OPCS (Office of Population Censuses and Surveys) (1991) *The Census*, London: HMSO.

Opie, A. (1994) 'The instability of the caring body: gender and caregivers of confused older people', *Qualitative Health Research*, vol 4, no 19, pp 31-50.

Orloff, A.S. (1993) 'Gender and the social rights of citizenship: the comparative analysis of gender relations and welfare states', *American Sociological Review*, vol 58, pp 303-28.

Ostner, I. (1993) 'Slow motion: women, work and the family in Germany', in J. Lewis (ed) *Women and social policies in Europe*, Aldershot: Edward Elgar.

Ostner, I. (1998) 'The politics of care policies in Germany', in J. Lewis (ed) *Gender, social care and welfare state restructuring in Europe*, Aldershot: Ashgate.

Pabst, St (1999) 'Mehr Arbeitsplätze für Geringqualifizierte nach Einführung der Pflegeversicherung? Beschäftigungswirkungen des SGB XI im ambulanten Bereich', Monatszeitschrift des Wirtschafts- und sozialwissenschaftlichen Instituts in der Heinz-Böckler-Stiftung (WSI-Mitteilungen), no 4, pp 234-40.

Parker, G. (1992) *With this body: caring and disability in marriage*, Buckingham: Open University Press.

Pateman, C. (1989) *The disorder of women*, Cambridge: Polity.

Peace, S., Kellaher, L. and Willcocks, D. (1997) *Re-evaluating residential care,* Buckingham: Open University Press.

Peirce, C.S. (1979) *Collected papers of Charles Sanders Peirce*, edited by C. Hartshorne and P. Weiss, vol 7, Cambridge, MA: Belknap Press.

Penrose, V. (1990) 'Vierzig Jahre SED-Frauenpolitik: Ziele, Strategien und Ergebnisse', *Frauenforschung*, vol 8, no 4, pp 60-77.

Perri 6 (1997) *Escaping poverty: From safety nets to networks of opportunity,* London: Demos.

Peukert, D. (1990) 'Wohlfahrtsstaat und Lebenswelt', in L. Niethammer et al (eds) *Bürgerliche Gesellschaft in Deutschland*, Frankfurt: Franz Fischer Verlag.

Phillips, J. (1996) 'The future of social work with older people in a changing world', in N. Parton (ed) *Social theory, social change and social work*, London: Routledge.

Philpott, T. (1994) *Managing to listen: A guide to user involvement for mental health services users,* London: King's Fund Centre.

Plaschke, J. (1984) 'Subsidiarität und "Neue Subsidiarität"', in R. Bauer and H. Diessenbacher (eds) *Organisierte Nächstenliebe: Wohlfahrtsverbände und Selbsthilfe in des Krise des Sozialstaats,* Opladen: Westdeutscher Verlag.

Pollack, D. (1992) 'Zwischen alten Verhaltens dispositionen und neuen Anforderungensprofilen – Bemerkungen zu den mentalitätsspezifischen Voraussetzungen des Operierens von Interessenverbänden und Organisationen in den neuen Bundesländern', *Probleme der Einheit,* vol 12, no 2, pp 489-508.

Pollack, D. and Pickel, G. (1998) 'Die ostdeutsche Identität – Erbe des DDR-Sozialismus oder Produkt der Wiedervereinigung? Die Einstellung der Ostdeutschen zu sozialer Ungleicheit und Demokratie', *Aus Politik und Zeitgeschichte,* B41-2, pp 9-23.

Putnam, D. (1993) *Making democracy work: Civic traditions in modern Italy,* Princeton: Princeton University Press.

Qureshi, H. and Walker, A. (1989) *The caring relationship: Elderly people and their families,* Basingstoke: Macmillan.

Ramon, S. (1998) 'Introduction', in S. Ramon, *The interface between social work and social policy,* Birmingham: British Association of Social Workers.

Ribbens, J. and Edwards, R. (1998) *Feminist dilemmas in qualitative research: Public knowledge and private lives,* London: Sage Publications.

Riemann, G. and Schütze, F. (1991) '"Trajectory" as a basic theoretical concept for analysing suffering and disorderly social processes', in D. Maines (ed) *Social organisation and social processes,* New York: de Gruyter.

Riley, D. (1988) *'"Am I that name?" Feminism and the category of "women" in history,* London: MacMillan.

Roller, E. (1992) *Einstellungen der Bürger zum Wohlfahrtsstaat der Bundesrepublik Deutschland,* Opladen: Westdeutscher Verlag.

Rosanvallon, P. (1988) 'The decline of social visibility', in J. Keane (ed) *Civil society and the state,* London: Verso.

Rosenhaft, E. and Lee, W. R. (1997) 'State and society in modern Germany – Beamtenstaat, Klassenstaat, Sozialstaat', in W. R. Lee and E. Rosenhaft (eds) *State, social policy and social change in Germany 1880-1994*, Oxford: Berg.

Rosenthal, G. (1993) 'Reconstruction of life stories. Principles of selection in generating stories for narrative biographical interviews', in R. Josselson and A. Lieblich (eds) *The narrative study of lives*, vol 3, London: Sage Publications.

Roth, G. (1999) 'Auflösung oder Konsolidierung korporatistischer Strukturen durch die Pflegeversicherung?', *Zeitschrift für Sozialreform*, vol 45, no 5, pp 418-47.

Royal Commission on Long-term Care (1999) *With respect to old age: Long-term care – rights and responsibilities*, London: HMSO.

Ruppel, F. and King, A. (1995) 'The German care insurance and British community care: comparative perspectives', *Social Work in Europe*, vol 2, no 1, pp 12-16.

Rustin, M. (1998) 'From individual life histories to sociological understanding', in *SOSTRIS Working Paper no 3, Case study material: Lone parents*, London: University of East London, Centre for Biography in Social Policy.

Sachße, C. and Tennstedt, F. (1980) *Geschichte der Armenfürsorge in Deutschland*, 2 vols, Stuttgart: Kohlhammer.

Scheff, T. (1997) *Emotions, the social bond and human reality: Part/whole analysis*, Cambridge: Cambridge University Press.

Schwartz, D. B. (1997) *Who cares? Rediscovering community*, Boulder, CO: Westview Press.

Seibel, W. (1989) 'The function of mellow weakness: non-profit organisations as problem non-solvers in Germany', in E. James (ed) *The non-profit sector in international perspective*, New York: Oxford University Press.

Shanin, T. (1998) 'Placing social work within social theory and political practice', in S. Ramon (ed) *The interface between social work and social policy*, Birmingham: British Association of Social Workers.

Shilling, C. (1997) 'The undersocialised conception of the embodied agent in modern sociology', *Sociology,* vol 31, no 4, pp 737-54.

Smith, R., Gaster, L., Harrison, L., Martin, L., Means, R. and Thistlethwaite, P. (1993) *Working together for better community care,* Bristol: University of Bristol, School for Advanced Urban Studies.

Somers, M. (1995) 'Narrating and naturalising civil society and citizenship theory: the place of political culture and the public sphere', *Sociological Theory,* vol 13, no 3, pp 229-74.

SOSTRIS Working Papers 1-9 (1997-99) London: University of East London, Centre for Biography in Social Policy.

Taylor-Gooby, P. (1991) 'Welfare state regimes and welfare citizenship', *Journal of European Social Policy,* vol 1, no 2, pp 93-106.

Thompson, D. (1995) 'Constructing the 'private' carer: daughters of reform?', in H. Dean (ed) *Parents' duties, children's debt: The limits of policy interventions,* Aldershot: Arena.

Timms, N. (1983) *Social work values: An enquiry,* London: Routledge and Kegan Paul.

Titmuss, R. (1975) *Social policy: An introduction,* London: Allen and Unwin.

Titterton, M. (1992) 'Managing threats to welfare: the search for a new paradigm of welfare', *Journal of Social Policy,* vol 21, no 1, pp 1-23.

Tönnies, F. (1955) *Community and association,* London: Routledge.

Trappe, H. (1995) 'Handlungsstrategien von Frauen unterschiedlicher Generationen zur Verbindung von Familie und Beruf und deren Beeinflussung durch sozialpolitische Rahmenbedingungen', in Zentrum für interdisziplinäre Frauenforschung der Humboldt-Universität Berlin (ed) *Unter Hammer und Zirkel: Frauenbiographien vor dem Hintergrund ostdeutscher Sozialisationserfahrungen,* Pfaffenweiler: Centaurus.

Tronto, J. (1993) *Moral boundaries: A political argument for an ethic of care,* London: Routledge.

Twigg, J. (1989) 'Models of carers: how do social care agencies conceptualise their relationship with informal carers?', *Journal of Social Policy,* vol 18, no 1, pp 53-66.

Twigg, J. and Atkin, K. (1994) *Carers perceived: Policy and practice in informal care*, London: HMSO.

Ungerson, C. (1983) 'Women and caring: skills, tasks and taboos', in E. Gamarnikow, D. Morgan, J. Purvis and D. Taylorson (eds) *The public and the private*, London: Heinemann.

Ungerson, C. (1987) *Policy is personal: Sex, gender and informal care*, London: Tavistock.

Ungerson, C. (1997) 'Social politics and the commodification of care', *Social Politics,* vol 4, no 3, pp 362-81.

Vester, M. (1993) 'Das Janusgesicht sozialer Modernisierung', *Aus Politik und Zeitgeschichte*, vols 26-7, pp 3-19.

Vester, M. (1994) 'Solidarität im Spagat. Umbrüche und sozialer Wandel in Ost- und Westdeutschland', in H-W. Meyer (ed) *Aufbrüche-Anstösse*, Cologne: Bund-Verlag.

von Clausewitz, C. (1968) (edited and translated by A. Rapoport) *On war*, Harmondsworth: Penguin.

Walker, A. (1994) 'Community care policy: from consensus to conflict', in J. Bornat, C. Pereira, D. Pilgrim and F. Williams (eds) *Community care: A reader,* Buckingham: Open University Press.

Watson, P. (1993) 'Eastern Europe's silent revolution: gender', *Sociology,* vol 27, no 3, pp 471-87.

Wengraf, T. (2000) 'Uncovering the general from within the particular. From contingencies to typologies in the understanding of cases', in P. Chamberlayne, J. Bornat and T. Wengraf (eds) *The turn to biographical methods in social sciences: Comparative issues and examples*, London: Routledge.

Wengraf, T. (2001) *Qualitative research interviewing: semi-structured and biographic narrative interviewing*, London: Sage Publications.

Wielgohs, J. (1993) 'Anflösung und Transformation der ostdeutschen Bürgerbewegung', *Deutschland Archiv*, vol 26, no 4, pp 426-35.

Wilkinson, R. (1996) *Unhealthy societies: The afflictions of inequality*, London: Routledge.

Williams, F. (1993) 'Women and the community', in J. Bornat, C. Pereira, D. Pilgrim and F. Williams (eds) *Community care: A reader,* Buckingham: Open University Press.

Williams, F., Popay, J. and Oakley, A. (eds) (1999) *Welfare research: A critical review*, London: UCL Press.

Willoughby, J. and Keating, N. (1991) 'Being in control: the process of caring for a relative with Alzheimer's disease', *Qualitative Health Research*, vol 1, no 1, pp 27-50.

Wilson, H.S. (1989) 'Family caregiving for a relative with Alzheimer's dementia: coping with negative choices', *Nursing Research*, vol 38, no 2, pp 94-8.

Young, B. (1994) 'Asynchronitäten der deutsch-deutschen Frauenbewegung', *Prokla*, vol 24, no 1, pp 49-63.

Zapf, W. (1986) 'Development, structure and prospects of the German social state', in N. Rose and R. Shiratori (eds) *The welfare state East and West*, Oxford: Oxford University Press.

Appendix 1: Gestalt theory and the biographical method

The interviews were analysed using the principles of the socio-biographical method.

The techniques developed for the analysis are based on an understanding of life stories as having a 'Gestalt'. Within this approach, the telling of a life story is an *act of narrative composition*, in which the life experiences are selected and related to each other to create a construction of biography (Fischer-Rosenthal, 2000). When people tell their life story, it can be seen as a re-evaluation of the past life experiences, based on the context of the present experience and reaching out into the future. People present a theory of their own lives: out of the infinite details of one's past, only those are included which present a 'picture' of a life course from a present perspective. As such, life-story accounts present a theory and history of the self, based on the selective recall of the past (Rosenthal, 1993; Wengraf, 2000).

The aim of the analysis is the reconstruction of the underlying 'rules' which govern the life-history account. The guiding principle is the comparison of the lived and told life story (see chapter one, Introduction). Both aspects of the life story are analysed separately, with no references between the two. It is through this analytic step that the inter-relationships between structural determinants and personal experiences can be brought into relief. Reconstruction of the life story thereby does not imply the subjective meaning of the individual, but it has an objective quality which exists outside the intentions of the narrator.

The analysis of lived and told life story

Abduction

The principle of analysis used in this method is that of *'abduction'*. Developed by Charles Sanders Peirce, it involves generating hypotheses contained in a given unit of empirical data, progressing to hypotheses as to the further developments and then testing these with the empirical outcome (Peirce, 1979). By formulating hypotheses about the other options available to a person within a particular historical and social context, the procedure reconstructs the range of possibilities open to the subject in a certain situation.

This analytical procedure is applied to each individual step of analysis, and the hypotheses that have been generated are tested in their plausibility at subsequent points of the process of analysis. This in part laborious procedure is aided substantially through the analysis of cases in a *group setting*, which was used extensively to bring analysis forward and test out hypotheses with the group (see also chapter one, Introduction).

Analytic steps

Technically, this part of the analysis involves the following three steps:

1. The *chronological analysis of the biographical data*.
2. A *thematic field analysis*, which attempts to uncover the structuring rules of the account. It analyses the dominant themes in the account, and the linguistic forms the account is embedded in: narration, description and argumentation. These can reveal what time perspective is taken over the told event, whether it is dramatically relived (narration), evaluated from a present perspective (argumentation), or simply described. Differences in the modes of narration set pointers for further analysis or indicate particularly important periods in the biography. In our project, we noted pauses and interruptions in the flow of stories as important indicators of significant events in the account.
3. Both steps are brought together in *the comparison of the case 'structure'*. The biographical data and narrated life-story analysis are used to formulate overarching themes about the inter-relationships between the narrated and lived life (Chamberlayne and Rustin, 1999, p 25). Through a detailed analysis of crucial text passages which relate to the emerging theories of the case structure (micro-analysis), the validity of these hypotheses is explored further and tested on the text. The comparison reveals the biographical context (how have events shaped and developed the person's orientation over the life course) and the present context of the narrated life story (what meaning these events have today). In the context of our use of case studies, we have been able to develop a biographical approach to caring experiences which reconstructs significant events in the development of the caring 'career' and carer strategies. In the analysis, the overall impact of the carer's biography, the understanding of self, and the way these have shaped the overall orientation to and perceptions of care, care work and care

relationships, are brought together to build up the case story of the carer. Although grounded in the life-world experiences of the individual person, the case studies present a highly interpreted and abstracted version of the person's actual experiences and life events, representing a sociological interpretation of the life world, which is used for purposes of illumination of more general social processes. Our reason for using the term 'case study' or 'case' when we talk about carers' accounts, rather than speaking more directly about the person, is to indicate the distance between the real individual and her or his history and our interpretation.

The themes, around which the main body of the book is structured, are the outcome of this final step of case analysis. The case studies themselves are the written-up case histories as produced by the socio-biographical method, and are used to illustrate the themes emerging from the comparisons (King and Chamberlayne, 1996).

Comparison of cases

Beyond the individual case

Above the level of the elaboration of each individual case reconstruction, in the last part of the analysis we move towards the comparison of cases, towards their insertion into a more comprehensive pattern of understanding and towards their simultaneous contribution to elaborating further, or rectifying, or even occasionally replacing such pre-existing larger theories.

The starting point of this process is the assertion that each individual case reveals much about the wholes of which it is part. Scheff (1997) has argued for relating, in Spinoza's phrase, "the smallest parts to the widest wholes":

> Extracts from discourse, one might argue, are microcosms, they contain within them, brief as they may be, intimations of the participants' origins in, and relations to, the institutions of the host society. (p 48)

However, the extraction or illumination of that connection requires knowledge and skill by the researcher-analyst. The notion of 'socio-biography' has been put forward to define the way in which the understanding of particular cases and their structural determinants in, and structuring effects on, their social matrix is built up. This occurs through the deployment of research and knowledge of more than the one particular case:

> We have to move beyond the self-understanding of social actors, which will unavoidably be limited by a particular life experience and set of cultural resources. Our aim is to bring to bear more generalised understandings, derived both from social science and from shared everyday knowledge of society, to situate and make sense of the individual experiences of subjects. (Rustin, 1998, p 113)

Commenting on the methodology within the SOSTRIS project, Rustin (1998) remarked:

> What we find ourselves doing is sketching in the relevant social context as we analyse each interview transcript, using the differences between them, what we may identify as previously established knowledge and the 'social knowledge' of our subjects, to fill out this picture.... The principal interpretive problem is to discern from the life-history narrative which are the relevant segments of social structure and culture which are 'in play' in a given case. That is, *both* what is the specific context which is shaping a life, *and* which social spaces are being remade, or reinvented by an individual.... These case studies lead us to the 'filling-out' of social structures and local cultures which are initially merely implicit and gestured towards in the narratives of our subjects.... We are not so much trying to 'map' our findings onto an existing sociology or social-policy scheme, as trying to develop from our case studies some kind of adequate 'map' on which they can be plotted. (Rustin, 1998, pp 114, 115, 118)

Towards generalisation

Individual cases are compared to other cases with similar and/or contrasting characteristics, allowing more general themes to emerge in such a comparison within or across societies. This is a complex task in which the analytical work moves towards the development of very grounded typologies, as the comparison of cases highlights both common and different features of the cases being studied. This shift from the exploration of apparently contingent patterns to a better understanding or construction of more generally formulated typologies is discussed in Wengraf (2000, 2001). Primarily faithful to the concerns of Glaser and

Strauss's (1967) schools of grounded theorising, this work necessarily also involves at a certain point the researchers cautiously investigating relevant general theorising or 'orienting concepts' (Layder, 1998) already put forward by other researchers or developed during the course of the particular research, and (even more cautiously) exploring how the emergent comparative patterns of similarity and difference of studied cases can be related creatively (and not reductively) to existing patterns and typologies formulated in terms of such orienting concepts.

This latter move is not a question of (statistical) generalisation because the number of cases studied and the mode of sampling them are virtually certain not to satisfy the conditions needed for such statistical inference. It is more a question of studying cases in great depth and in their elaborated contexts so as to understand all cases better, and to improve the conceptual model for the description and understanding of all such cases. One might sum it up by saying that (statistical) generalisation is not possible from our cases but (conceptual) universalisation is.

Appendix 2: List of carers interviewed

The 76 interviewees are listed alphabetically, according to country. The case studies discussed in the main body of the text are highlighted in italics.

Interviewees in Bremen, West Germany

Name	Carer's age	Relationship (and age) of cared-for-person	Carer's recent occupation
Frau Alexander	*35*	*child (son 11)*	*housewife*
Frau Belling	56	child (daughter 23)	housewife
Frau Böttcher	35	child (son 3)	nurse
Herr Dumke	30	child (son 3) – adopted	care worker in residential home
Frau Franke	57	child (son 28)	laundry worker
Herr Hackmann	76	wife (about 74)	pensioner
Frau Hamann	*34*	*child (2)*	*medical doctor – not working*
Frau Hegemann	*43*	*husband (42)*	*bank worker*
Frau Igel	44	mother (about 70)	office worker – not working
Frau Jahn	60	mother (92)	pensioner
Frau Jakob	*59*	*husband (60)*	*cleaner*
Frau Luchtig	*55*	*mother (81)*	*shop worker – not working*
Frau and	*31*	*child*	*social worker – not working*
Herr Mahler	*30*	*(foster daughter 5)*	
Herr Nolte	55	mother (81)	business consultant
Frau Otto	84	husband (90)	pensioner
Frau Peters	25	child (foster son 1)	social work student
Frau Planck	35	child (son 2)	housewife
Frau Riese	67	husband (70)	housewife
Frau Rose	51	aunt (80)	secretary
Frau Schuhmann	32	child (son 7)	housewife
Frau Sommer	32	child (son 1)	housewife
Frau Sonne	41	father (84)	cleaner
Frau Walther	35	child (son 16)	cleaner
Frau Wegner	55	child (son 21)	housewife
Frau Werther	43	husband (47)	chemical engineer – not working
Herr Wolter	52	mother (82)	sailor – recently retired

Interviewees in Leipzig, East Germany

Name	Carer's age	Relationship (and age) of cared-for-person	Carer's recent occupation
Frau Arndt	23	*child (son 3)*	*trainee police officer*
Frau Bauer	30	child (son 2)	trainee business administrator
Frau Becker	80	husband (86)	retired
Frau Blau	61	*husband (62)*	*retired*
Frau Bredel	50	mother (84)	secretary
Herr and Frau Broch	63 60	mother (92)	retired
Frau Carlson	35	child (son 13)	technician
Frau Fäller	52	child (son 23)	care worker
Herr Fuchs	60	wife (59)	lecturer
Herr and Frau Grossmann	36 33	child (daughter 12)	trainee psychotherapist and medical doctor
Herr and Frau Grün	*31* *25*	*child (son 7)*	*parson* *nurse*
Frau Gutes	34	mother (55)	full-time carer
Frau Hager	59	mother (90)	invalidity pensioner
Frau Hildebrand	*37*	*child (daughter 14)*	*teacher*
Herr and Frau Koch	55 50	his mother (77)	secretary unemployed
Herr Krüger	70	wife (44)	retired
Frau Meissner	*41*	*child (daughter 20)*	*care worker*
Frau Pontek	37	child (son 13)	homeworker, unemployed
Frau Pusch	43	husband (53)	psychiatric nurse
Frau Richter	48	child (daughter 19)	care worker/nurse
Frau Riedel	41	mother (86)	educational/art therapist
Frau Roth	40	child (son 14)	office clerk
Frau Schubert	60	husband (58)	tool maker
Herr Schulz	59	mother (81)	early retired
Herr Speyer	*65*	*wife (57)*	*semi-retired taxi driver*
Frau Winter	56	child (son 31)	care worker

Interviewees in Britain

Name	Carer's age	Relationship (and age) of cared-for-person	Carer's recent occupation
East London Borough			
Mrs Baltic	46	son (18) husband (71)	housewife
Mrs Blake	47	son (25)	housewife
Mrs Buckley	54	daughter (20)	variety of jobs – not working
Mr Darrant	52	mother (88)	engineer
Mrs Elliot	60	grandson (29)	home machinist
Ms Graham	26	sister (22)	unemployed
Mr Horton	85	wife (74)	pensioner
Ms Hulme	63	friend (66)	pensioner
Mr Merton	42	wife (31)	variety of jobs – not working
Ms Murdoch	53	mother (78)	administrator
Mrs Poole	50	daughter (27)	nurse
Mrs Rajan	32	son (12)	housewife
Mr Scott and Mr Scott	61 67	brother (64)	pensioners
North London Borough			
Mr Allahm	65	wife (64)	retired
Mrs Bally	69	child (son 29)	retired
Mrs Bianco	28	daughter (3)	housewife
Mrs Carter	59	daughter (25)	housewife
Mrs Frost	45	husband (53)	housewife
Mrs Goodman	59	mother (81)	retired
Mrs Keith	27	child (son 5)	secretary – not employed
Ms Leonardi	51	mother (90)	secretary – not employed
Mr Morris	72	wife (68)	retired
Mrs Rossiter	47	mother (77)	shop assistant
Mrs Rushton	62	husband (60)	housewife

Index

Main references to case studies are in **bold** type.